EVERY
BODY
HOLDS
A STORY

Paperback ISBN 978-1-7782150-1-8
eBook ISBN 978-1-7782150-0-1

Edited by Cassie Jeans & Sue Ruhe
Book Designed by Doris Chung
Cover Designed by Michelle Fairbanks
eBook by Ellie Sipilä

Printed in North America

EVERY BODY HOLDS A STORY

A COLLABORATIVE BOOK SERIES WITH
SUE RUHE & MARSHA VANWYNSBERGHE

Contents

Author Bios

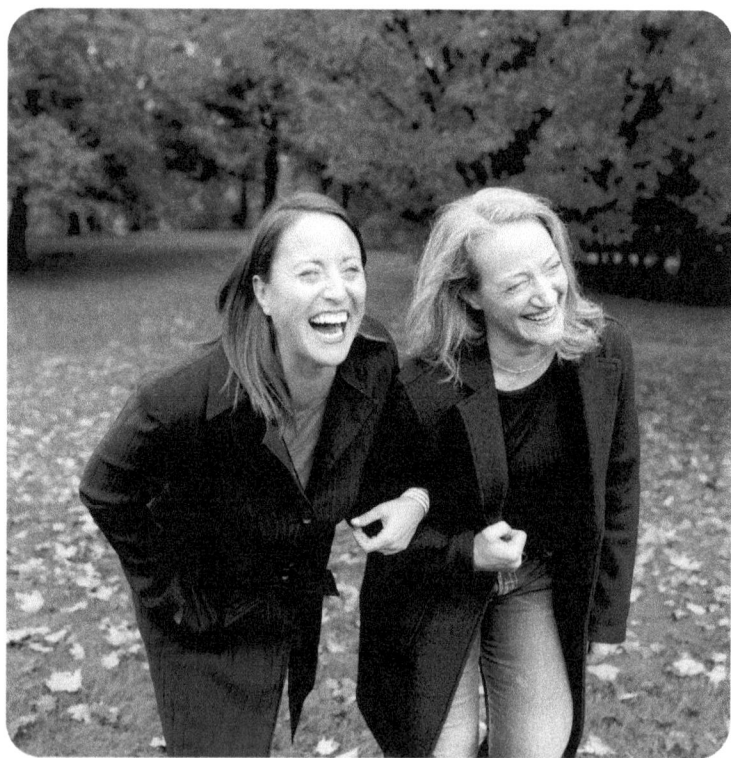

(Que intro music)

M: *"Hi, I'm Marsha Vanwynsberghe and I teach people how to own and change their stories to create a massive impact in the world."*

S: *"And I'm Sue Ruhe. I help people release those stories that they are holding onto at the cellular level."*

M: *"Together, as two podcasters and friends, we have created this space to share human body experiences from people who have shifted their stories from the inside out."*

S: *"Because Every Body. . ."*

M: *"Holds a story!"*

(outro music)

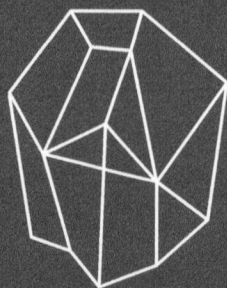

Introduction

In August 2020, this phrase pulsed through my body as my hands lay embedded in Marsha's abdominal fascia.

Every body holds a story.
Every body holds a story.

"What is this?" I thought, as I closed my eyes to focus. My hands burned as I continued to listen.

Our cells are magnificent structures. Holding us together while keeping the score. Everything we have ever endured, conquered, and created throughout our existence, gifts us our stories, that remain forever imprinted in our DNA.

Marsha and I often joke about how her body holds fifty-thousand stories. From Immunocompromised conditions to multiple miscarriages, to countless surgeries—her body has been through the wringer! How is she still breathing? How is she still walking? How is she still doing everything she does every day?

This concept that *every body* holds a story came to life immediately following her treatment that day. It started as a Podcast and grew into something more. We wanted to create a platform for people to share their stories. A space to share human body experiences that inspire, educate and support and as a collection that could be left on this earth for future generations. Each one of us holds a myriad of experiences, from before and within the womb, bringing us to the exact place we are in right now. The stories you are about to read are real-life experiences from people who want to help and support others and to offer insight and resources for anyone who may be navigating similar circumstances. We are beyond proud of these authors for how they share themselves vulnerably while offering support and solutions that will help others on their journeys.

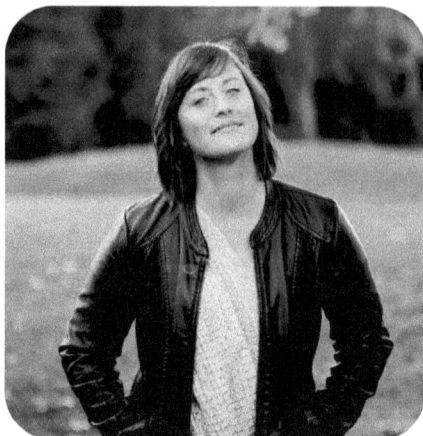

Sue Ruhe

Sue Ruhe B.A., R.M.T., is an Intuitive Myofascial Release Therapist of 15 years. Her work has helped clients shift restricted areas found within their fascial matrix, to create more fluidity and alignment within the body. In addition, she has been able to help her clients overcome the anxiety they unknowingly hang onto, so that they can move beyond it.

In 2020, Sue transitioned her in-person practice to the virtual space where she now guides clients with connecting their hands into their own fascia, to help reduce stress, anxiety, and other body pain. Sue is an author, podcaster, and proud mother. She resides in London Ontario Canada, with her partner and 10-year-old daughter. Her mission has always been to help guide the next generation in achieving a better understanding of these bodies we have been given.

IG @_sueruhe

CHAPTER ONE

Healing and Trust Go Hand in Hand

Marsha Vanwynsberghe

I roll over and my clock says 5:00 am.

Ugh, seriously?!

Could be worse, some days it's 3:00 am and I didn't even get to wake up to my birds. Yes, I have an alarm clock that wakes me up gradually to the sounds of nature, birds and sunlight. I go to sleep to nature sounds and a deep red light that is supposed to improve my quality of sleep. I practice breathwork in the morning and before I go to sleep. It all works, just not every day. I might as well get up, I'm awake now.

Starting my day with a litre of water (yes I said that), lemon water, a pre-workout, adaptogen tea, the second tea of lion's mane, mixed with my MCT oil, honey, nootropics, then my sludge water of green juice, vitamin C, collagen, electrolytes and my slew of vitamins. I fill my gallon water bottle and know that I will likely drink 1.5 gallons almost every day.

Nighttime routines include my gold turmeric tea, magnesium, meditation, breathwork, reading, feeling my gratitudes, writing my celebrations or listening to a meditation or hypnosis. No joke, this routine is as custom as my morning routine. I am not a doctor or nutritionist, but I have spent years working on my best combo in regards to what I need to feel my best to give myself a fighting chance before my day even starts.

Some days I journal, meditate, do breathwork, read ten pages of whatever I have on the go, or I brain dump and write out ideas because my head is constantly swirling with ideas. I go inward and listen to what I need that day for movement. The type of movement is optional, and it can range from mobility work, barbell work, circuit training or stretching. Every day involves non-negotiable five to six-kilometre walks with my dog Izzy, trust me when I say non-negotiable.

As I reflect on the last twenty years and twelve surgeries including a full hysterectomy and back surgery that left me with so much titanium, I am acutely aware of how important and necessary movement is for my body, brain, mental and emotional health. I have been committed to my health in all aspects for so many years I wonder where I'd be if I wasn't this committed. As my friend and co-lead author Sue says, "I probably wouldn't be here if I didn't fight for my health or make it the priority that it is."

After experiencing a partial molar pregnancy in 2002, I began a new trajectory of consciously choosing to make my health my number one priority. I remember sitting in the doctor's office after my D&C (my 4th miscarriage) and being told it was a partial molar pregnancy. This was a 1 in 100,000 odds, and very rare. The word "rare" became a trigger for me over the years because I can't count the number of times this word was spoken to me with regards to my health. After the D&C, the mass results came back benign after six weeks of waiting and being told what the treatment would look like if it was cancerous. Worry, dread, fear and lack of control led to trust, faith, and belief that my story wasn't over yet. This is after two years of monthly hormone testing, followed by six total years of hormone medications and multiple exploratory surgeries including ablation and burning of endometrial tissue. No one talked about endometriosis at this time, and I am sure I had this condition all my life. After six years of fighting for my health and multiple surgeries, I made the executive decision to ask for a full hysterectomy. This came from a vision I had on Christmas Eve 2007 when a voice said, "If you don't push for a hysterectomy, then this will be your last Christmas." This message was clear as day and ironically the word "hysterectomy" had never even been mentioned before this moment. But (and if you know me you know I rarely use this word) I was so burnt out, exhausted, and drained of the possibility of repeating this cycle of one to two surgeries per year. I was turning thirty-eight years old, and I couldn't fight this way any longer. I was at a turning point and mentally was giving up hope. I told my OB (obstetrician) I wanted a full hysterectomy. He laughed and stated, "Not a chance," he said, "you're far too young." Deep down I knew this had to happen. Call it gut instinct or a note from a higher power but I knew I couldn't mentally or physically continue the way I was.

I fought so hard for a procedure I knew nothing about, and it scared me to be pushed into full menopause in a two-hour timespan when most women have a decade for their bodies to adjust. I knew in my gut I had to push this to happen with no clue why, but my inner fighter told me to push. It took a lot of convincing, determination and pushing to have the hysterectomy done. Right before my surgery, my OB said,

"We'll keep your ovaries." I said, "Nope, I guarantee my ovaries are the problem." He asked me if I wanted to make a bet and I said, "Sure, you're on." When I woke up in the recovery room, my OB looked at me and asked, "How did you know?" I smiled in my groggy state replying, "I just knew." I will never forget his words, "I am not sure you would have made it to forty without this surgery." I took a breath, smiled, and knew I made the right decision. This was the beginning of learning to listen to my intuition and letting it guide me.

Part of the fear of making critical decisions is not knowing the outcome ahead of time. I can't count the number of times people have asked me that question, "How did you know it was the right decision?" I didn't, and in many ways, we never do when we're asked to have faith. All we can do is choose to stay where we are or make a decision to walk into the unknown.

It's in these moments I recognize and embrace my fighter side. I know I wouldn't be where I am today and wouldn't have overcome so many challenges (health, personal and emotional) if I didn't have this fighter characteristic. I have learned to embrace her (my fighter side) qualities, love on them and understand she is the reason I have come this far. However, there comes a point where we all learn that our strengths can eventually become our weaknesses. The fighter brought me to one key point in my life and couldn't take me any further. She still shows up regularly because she is my default but what I am referring to is the turning point while I was in the hospital, recovering from back surgery in October 2020 when I experienced a lightbulb moment. I realized the fighter side was not the characteristic I needed to heal and move

In surrendering, I slowly learned how to trust.

forward. I had done it this way for so long and I was beyond exhausted from the cycle of pushing and fighting, I knew I had to surrender to a different way of living because it was the only option I had left. In surrendering, I slowly learned how to trust. This was a big and scary word to a woman who spent her life fighting. I honestly didn't have any other options and I am grateful it unfolded in this manner. This was the moment I committed to my healing, I listened to what my body needed, and I truly honoured her for bringing me this far. I created morning and evening routines, work schedules, stacked habits and got curious about what I needed every single day. Instead of pushing the boulder uphill and resenting the challenges and experiences, I decided to step aside, leave it behind and walk forward. I checked in regularly, asked what I needed and then followed through. Not just for my body and health, for my business, for my relationships, for my energy, boundaries, self-care, literally everything. This became the game-changer in my life, health and business and I never would have learned these lessons without spending years as a fighter. I didn't do it wrong, I did it exactly as I was supposed to and for that, I am damn proud of myself.

Where can you honour your body, your soul, the fighter, the traits, and the characteristics that brought you to this point in your life? Where can you stop resenting the thought of, you didn't do it right, or that you're not enough, and instead love all the messy parts of yourself as who you are? You cannot love yourself and hate all the experiences that make you who you are. It just doesn't work that way. Learning to love yourself means embracing the gifts in the challenges and always remembering someone somewhere is praying for the solutions you are holding onto.

Creating this platform with my dear friend Sue, interviewing so many incredible guests on the Every Body Holds A Story Podcast, and working closely with the author's stories you are about to read, including a very special chapter written by my sister, makes me so proud of her alongside all the incredible authors. This became possible because the fighter kept me alive and directed me to Sue, and together our work brought us to this point in our lives. A point where we support and share stories of incredible humans in the upcoming chapters. I know our vision is just starting and we are beyond proud and grateful that these women raised their hands and stepped forward to share their stories with you.

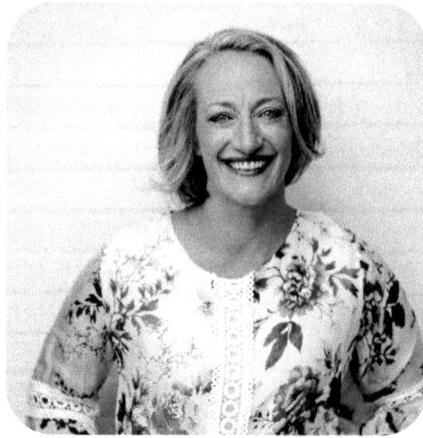

Marsha Vanwynsberghe

Storytelling Business Coach, Speaker, Author & Podcaster. Marsha is the 6-time Bestselling author of, "When She Stopped Asking Why." She shares her lessons as a parent who dealt with teen substance abuse that tore her family unit apart. Marsha has been published six times in collaborative books including, "Owning Your Choices," sharing inspiring stories of courage from women around the world. Through her tools, NLP certifications, programs, coaching, and two podcasts, Marsha teaches the power of Radical Responsibility and Owning Your Choices in your life. She empowers women how to own and stand on their stories, be conscious leaders, and build platform businesses that create massive impact.

IG @marshavanw | FB @marshavanwynsberghe

I dedicate this chapter to my incredible husband, Brad, and to all the amazing girlfriends, family members, and mentors who supported me over the years. I am grateful for all of the friends who were there for me unconditionally whom I learned how to ask for help and allow in. I learned to value myself, appreciate my worthiness, and receive the support of others. I am especially grateful for the people who helped me to heal and recover from my back surgery in 2020. Sue Ruhe was one of those people who helped me to heal, breathe and support myself as I prepared for this surgery and recovered over the next few months. We came into each other's lives at a very key time and I know the universe knew what I needed. This difficult time was the beginning of Every Body Holds A Story, the podcast, and this book you are now reading. I am also thankful for my intuition and faith for guiding me through. I am here today, alive and well because of them. I also want to thank my boys for being my best teachers. They have taught me how to love, accept, forgive and truly live in gratitude for the moments I used to take for granted.

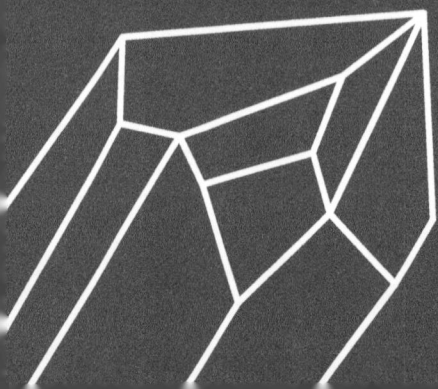

CHAPTER TWO

The Hero Who Inspired Me

Charlene Freeman

One of my greatest accomplishments in life happens to be saving a life. Although it may sound like an accomplishment, it is not a story I like to share. I have kept this experience a deep secret that I have only shared with my closest friends and immediate family. Unlike other people who are afraid of sharing negative experiences, I am afraid of sharing my experience to avoid experiencing criticism and making my decision feel small in my own eyes.

When I decided to make a living donation, I was only focused on saving a life. One factor I did not consider was the additional effects that come with the donation of an organ. Before the procedure, one is educated on the living donation program; however, no one can prepare you for the social effects the donation has on your life. For example, many people do not know a lot about the living donation program. Anytime I share my story on donation to create awareness, I feel I will be judged or seen as an attention seeker. Every time someone has known I am a living donor, they have reacted towards me as a hero, a reaction

I do not prefer. When I decided to be a living donor, I didn't do it for heroism or praise, but I knew I had a responsibility to educate, advocate and create awareness for organ donation and its importance to society. Most people do not know it exists, and sadly, it is not something they learn about until serious illness touches someone they love. I hope that someone will read my story and find a personal call to themselves to reach out for more information and perhaps if the time is right, for them to become a living donor.

My journey to organ donation began eleven years ago when I had a front-row seat to watch my uncle battling end-stage liver disease. It was hard to see a loved one suffer significantly and I was horrified by the thought that if nothing were done, he would die in front of our eyes. The feeling of helplessness that comes with disease worsens when one understands their loved one does not have long to live. However, before the transplant, we faced an obstacle in the form of a long wait on the transplant list.

During our wait, his health deteriorated daily; he was dying before our eyes. We were helpless and hopeless, as there was nothing we could do to save our uncle. An even harder dilemma was being told he was not yet sick enough to be put to the top of the list, which seemed hard to believe. Secretly, I remember hoping he would get worse so he would be moved to the top for the best chance of getting a donor. The moral dilemma of wanting him to get worse could result in him being too sick to receive a transplant even if one was found. It became a balancing act of thoughts and emotions that were a part of us every second of the day. The world seemed to stand still, the clock could not tick fast enough, and I wondered how the rest of the world could carry on as if everything was normal.

A few weeks later, he was moved to the top of the list, where we all prayed he would one day get that lifesaving phone call, his second chance at life. The heartache was unbearable. Watching so much pain in my aunt's face, she was about to lose the love of her life, my cousin would lose her father and my dad was about to lose his best friend. All we could do was watch, wait and pray, knowing the longer the wait, the slimmer the chance of him surviving.

I will never forget the day I received the phone call from my father to inform me our miracle had happened; he was an 'acceptable' match with a deceased donor, the result of a tragic accident. For the first time, the reality of the situation resonated with me. While my family had their prayers answered and were given the golden ticket of hope, no one seemed to realize the cost of saving my uncle. My family received a miracle at the expense of another family losing their loved one.

Throughout the entire process, I had never given organ donation much thought to where the organ would come from, other than the fact it was my uncle's ticket to a second chance at life. My miracle had somehow become someone else's tragedy. The thought of it made me feel sick, how the answer to our family's prayers could be at the expense of someone else. Ultimately, someone had to die for our miracle to happen. One second, I was elated with hope and the next second with utter disappointment of the situation. The irony of it stayed with me long after his physical recovery and I found I was thinking more and more about donations.

This propelled me to research ways I could pay it forward; I felt called to action. It didn't take me long to find the living donor organ transplant program out of the Toronto General Hospital, and I was horrified to find that all along there was a living liver donation program.

The Ajmera Transplant Centre at the University Health Network's Toronto Hospital specializes in saving people with heart failure, diabetes, kidney disease, lung disease and liver cancer. The program is the largest in North America and is equipped with the right team of specialists and technology to help patients. The facility cares for over 700 patients annually and has completed over 6000 organ transplants. The facility continuously conducts studies to improve its quality of care and increase the number of patients they help annually. While the program is doing great work, it mainly has to rely on organ transplants from donations from dying or dead donors. Living donations have been a viable and potential way of contributing to other people's lives and can help expand the organization's work. I learned that my uncle did not have to wait for a deceased donor to get a second chance at life. Any one of us could have stepped up to be tested to be his donor. A tragedy did not have to happen for a miracle to occur.

During the time of my uncle's illness, I felt powerless and ignorant to the fact I could have been proactive and explored potential solutions, only to be astonished that there was a potential solution all along. All those weeks he lost in the hospital, clinging to his life, suffering and in pain, would have changed if one of us had stepped up to be his donor. During that time, we took a front-row seat watching his body fail and suffer and we could have helped. I do not know if I would have been a match for my uncle as I know there are strict criteria that need to match but I could have tried. I was unaware and he never asked. Why didn't he ask? His answer, "I came to peace with dying, the only thing worse than dying is knowing that I was putting someone I love at risk and I would never do that." At that moment, I knew he was one of the strongest people I had ever known. He loved everyone unconditionally and was not willing to risk anyone's life for the chance to save his own. A person's true character is not measured in the highs of life, but rather, it's found in the lows. Facing death every day, not knowing how many days you have left, and being at peace with that is remarkable. In my eyes, he was the true hero; he had the courage and strength to believe in his journey without any anger or resentment. I could feel the dilemma he had and I understood his situation.

Morally, I had a hard time accepting all of it. I somehow felt the world was out of balance; it was a liver short. If I had stepped up for my uncle, the deceased donor could have gone to save someone else's life. I felt the need and the obligation to pay that forward, no matter what that meant for me. I spent much time talking with my husband and four children about how I felt and what I wanted to do. They were supportive of my idea and agreed to walk the journey with me. They whole-heartedly lifted me up, understood what I wanted to do, and gave me their blessing to move forward.

I reached out to the living donor program, filled out their application to become a donor, and waited for the journey to begin. Within a week, the program contacted me to explain the next steps. The first step was a barrage of preliminary tests to be performed at the hospital in Toronto. The tests would determine if I was in good health to be considered a donor. That first appointment was when I met my doctor, head coordinator of the living donation program. Rarely in my life have I come across an individual who can put me at ease so effortlessly. He went over my initial blood work and tests and confirmed I was a good candidate but needed to understand my reasoning for wanting to be a donor. After a long discussion, I knew I was put on the donor path to meet him; he listened to my journey and conveyed his support and blessing moving forward. He explained while one may be emotionally ready to be a donor, one needs to understand the consequences and risks of donation.

He explained that the surgery would take 6-8 hours, have a six-week recovery time, and was considered major surgery with a 0.2 to 0.5% risk of major complications. The procedure could be considered a low-risk, high-reward procedure because of its potential to save lives. Liver donation does not affect a person's life expectancy, especially if an individual continues to live a healthy life. Although research is limited in this area, there are no significant risks or consequences known yet. He suggested donating a kidney instead due to the reduced risk and easier surgery, however, I quickly refused as I needed to follow through with the liver donation, no matter what risks that brought.

From there, it was a whirlwind. I was admitted to the hospital for a few days so they could accomplish a number of tests at once, rather than having me travel back and forth. I shared a room with a woman waiting for a liver who was very open with her story. She shared that twenty years ago, she donated a portion of her liver to her sister, to save her life. However, years later started to get sick herself and now needed a liver. She had lived both sides of giving and needing and had the unique perspective of understanding my journey, perhaps more than anyone else had or could. She did caution me on questions for my well-being, but understood the call I felt to pay it forward. She was instrumental when the head of surgery came to meet with me. She listened and asked the questions she knew I needed the answers for, while he sat patiently answering them all, talking to both of us for long periods on several occasions. There was no doubt in my mind they were put on my path for a reason, and I would be forever grateful to them.

Without hope, we have nothing.

My last evaluation was a psychological assessment with a social worker. She prepared me for the 'what-ifs' involved in the procedure. She prepared and asked me questions about all possible situations. What if there were complications and the transplant was not successful for the recipient and me? What if the recipient did not survive? How would I feel? How would I cope with this? Would I blame myself? These questions were critical in making my final decision. I gave this much thought and determined; what I was offering was hope. The same 'hope' we prayed for when my uncle was waiting for a donor. That hope was all I was in control of, the outcome I could not control. Without hope, we have nothing.

I was discharged from the hospital and cleared for donation; the doctors then searched for the recipient. They told me they had to match my physical build to match either a small female or an older child and asked pointedly if I had a preference. I wanted my donation to go to someone who needed it the most. My only condition was not to donate to someone who needed a liver due to his/her own life choices. I firmly believe everyone deserves a second chance; but that was not my issue. I wanted my donation to go to someone who had no choice, and the illness was out of their control. My uncle did not smoke or drink, he led a healthy lifestyle, which did also factor into my decision regarding the recipient. The process took a month before another doctor contacted me. They had selected a recipient, the recipient had been notified, and the surgery date had been set.

On August 29, 2012, I underwent major surgery to donate 60% of my liver as an anonymous living donor to a single mother. I would be lying if I said I was not scared. I was terrified but knew I needed to have the same conviction and strength my uncle had demonstrated for years. I was admitted into the ICU the night before surgery where I spent a sleepless night wondering if I had made the right decision.

My family accompanied me to the hospital, their presence was my strength. They gave me the conviction to continue down the journey I started months ago. I knew they were terrified for me, but I did not see that on their faces. They were pinnacles of strength and support. On the morning of the surgery the doctors allowed my husband, mother, and two of my children to come with me to the pre-op area when they prepared me for surgery. I was not prepared for all of the machines, IV lines and other contraptions they hooked me up to while my family watched. I was also not prepared for the looks of terror on each of their faces when the doctor came over to tell them it was time to say goodbye, and that they were taking me to the operating room. The tears were overwhelming and for the first time I saw the raw terror in each of their faces and I knew I had overlooked what my journey meant for everyone else, the sacrifice they all were forced to make.

After the surgery, my first memory was waking up in the ICU with the three incredible doctors at my bedside who held my hand and gave me the news that the surgery was successful and said, "Today, you were the hero of another family's story." Those words have stayed with me and have lifted me up over the years when I've felt low. Those powerful words remind me of my bravery. My uncle made sure to let me know I had done something someone will never forget as long as they live.

The week recovering in the hospital was humbling for me. My pain felt real, but little in comparison to those around me. While I was there recovering from elective surgery, knowing I would recover, I was surrounded by others who were waiting for their miracle to happen. Their lives were hanging in limbo. I imagined the pain they were in, just like my uncle had been. I imagined how much pain they felt and how long they would continue to be in pain if they soon did not receive a donation. I could not imagine living every second of life waiting for a miracle you desperately needed. The uncertainty over the next day, week and month was what made the pain worse. Talking to my roommate before my surgery, she told me she questioned where she had gone wrong, what she had done wrong, and how long she had to wait. My doctor had also told me that the process of matching donor and recipient was complicated because it had to be a perfect match. Failing to find a perfect match meant the recipient's body might reject the liver. Once the liver has been donated to someone else, it can no longer be used for another. If the matches were not perfect, then all the work would have been for nothing.

My family gave me the encouragement and support I needed. My husband was my lifeline. He stayed by my side the entire week, days spent at my bedside and nights spent at the hotel across the street. I could not have asked for more from my family. I wanted their support and acceptance of my decision during the process, but I did not stop to think of how it affected them. That remains my only regret. Although the surgery was considered safe, it was still major surgery and carried risks; those risks burdened my family because they also had a sacrifice to make. I should have considered how they felt about the risk I was taking. I should have taken the time to carry them along my journey and ensure they were as prepared emotionally, physically, and mentally as I was.

It was hard on them and there is a difference when a healthy individual chooses to have elective major surgery. It is a hurdle for surgeons as well because they are sworn to do no harm but ultimately are putting the life of a healthy individual at risk. My family will never truly understand how grateful I am to them, as they are a large part of saving a life; in reality, they helped save the recipients and mine. Without their support, I would not have been able to make this sacrifice.

After I was discharged from the hospital, I spent a lot of time reflecting on the journey and examining why it took a tragedy in my life to educate me on becoming a donor. Why was I so ignorant of the pain and suffering happening around me? Why aren't more people stepping up to help those in need? *The realization that the value we place on our loved ones' lives is greater than our value on a stranger.* This is a natural and obvious statement; however, it occurred to me that this value is a piece of what is missing in the world. Should we not be willing to help our neighbours in need, as easily as we would help our loved ones? They are someone's loved ones. Just because they are not ours' does not make them unworthy of our help. Organ donation is not on anyone's radar until it becomes personal. Once it becomes personal, it becomes a race against time and one where you'll do everything in your power to find help. That is the moment when you see life differently. This change of lens is where my journey to organ donation began. While my family had suffered for a long time, I did not want other families to go through the same and I could choose to do something about that.

I turned my attention toward advocacy, not only to organ donation but also to the living donor program. I believe organ donation should be a person's choice, also one they should be made aware of. People sign their donor cards with good intentions and believe they know about the program, but they don't have all the information. Many more people are willing to donate their organs but do not know enough to start the journey. Not everyone can put their own lives on hold to help someone else, especially someone they do not know, but there are people out there who can. When I started my journey, I had my own established business; I was financially secure and had my family's support. Essentially everything I needed I had, so the timing was right. All I aimed to do was get the word out there so that people in that ideal position would stop to think about it and possibly decide to help if they could. Or at most, educate others so they knew it was a possibility. I sadly felt paralyzed, unable to deliver my message because it required me to tell my story, which I was unable to do.

A couple of years ago, Toronto General Hospital reached out to me during organ donor month to help advocate. They wanted to interview me for their website, do a photo shoot for their billboards and go on live radio to tell my story. The problem for me was self-disclosure. I could not advocate anonymously. What they were asking would require me to speak out, call attention to my personal decision and put it out there for comments from others. My family did not even know the hospital had a billboard of my face on display at their front entrance every April. As suspected, there were negative comments regarding my 'anonymous donation' but not a public campaign. The criticism again shut me down, made me feel small, and my reason for donating small.

Why does doing something nice for a stranger result in shame and speculation from people we do not know? It is difficult to break the barrier between advocacy for helping those in need and skepticism of others, believing there had to be more to gain than just paying forward a good deed. I agree I did get personal satisfaction from paying my uncle's transplant forward and the unmeasurable pride in myself for doing something to help someone in need. Therefore, this story is more than just advocacy; owning my decisions, being proud of them and not apologizing for wanting to bring awareness to a program few know exists.

I still have unanswered questions to this day. Such as, why does the concept of paying it forward happen only if someone does something nice, to begin with? Who starts the process? How do we get people to step up more often and help others in need with no return expected or required? What is required to shift the mindset to want to help unconditionally when people are in need? These questions may remain unanswered for a long time because there are no real candid answers on why people do not help unconditionally. It is essentially the concept of psychological egoism in place, which many are adamant to accept. People have not internalized the concept of helping others without conditions or expectations, which ultimately is the very reason why my journey to liver donation is met with skepticism. Perhaps a solution is to stop the label *anonymous* donor and people should refrain from asking *who* the recipient was to make it more socially acceptable. Donating to a loved one is considered expected while donating to a stranger is considered heroic. Shouldn't they be considered the same?

My journey of donation has changed me. It has broadened my lens of compassion from my loved ones only, to everyone. I know I cannot change the world, but I did change the world for one person. This is where the ripple begins.

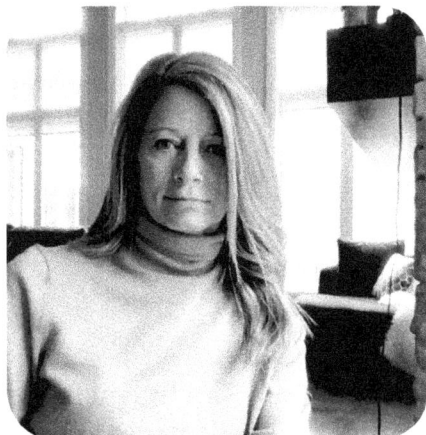

Charlene Freeman

As a dynamic business leader and advocate for organ donation, Charlene Freeman has a deep passion for personal growth and professional development. She has a knack for helping others and has dedicated her life to doing so in any capacity. Charlene is an active member of the Sunshine Foundation, an organization dedicated to answering the dreams of chronically ill, seriously ill, physically challenged and abused children from ages three to eighteen. Here, she orchestrated and executed a charity fundraiser to secure $40,000 in donations. Charlene has also actively supported the Salvation Army's Adopt a Family Campaign for ten years. She is currently the President and CEO of I.M.A. Inventory Management Analysis, a global, multi-million-dollar organization, guiding all operations and overseeing twenty-four personnel. Outside of work, volunteering and advocating for organ donation, Charlene enjoys spending time with her husband, four children, and two grandchildren.

I dedicate this chapter to my husband Jason and my children, Kaitlyn, Emily, Brooke, and Jordan, for all their unconditional and unwavering love and support. Thank you for being my biggest cheerleader, always being in my corner, and believing in me when I lost belief in myself. To my uncle who taught me the true meaning of heroism and inspired me to forever pay it forward. Your words, your stoicism, and your bravery will forever inspire me. Thank you to my parents for their love and support in all the good and bad times, you taught me the true meaning of family. Thank you to my sister Marsha for giving me this platform, guidance, and courage to tell my story. Lastly, I want to express my sincere gratitude to all of the doctors and nurses at the Ajmera Transplant Centre at Toronto General Hospital. Your expert guidance, care, and compassion will never be forgotten.

CHAPTER THREE

Human **DO**ing vs Human **BE**ing

Peggy Birr

"Hey Peggy, do you have a minute?"

My inside voice screams "*No*", but of course, I will help. I set down my k-basin of IV and blood draw supplies that are ordered for my patients. Teamwork is how we (and patients), survive in the ER.

"Peggy, I put someone in bed five." I hear the triage nurse call out.

As I proceed to help my colleague, I notice two of my patients ringing their bells and a third one is calling out, "*Nurse, Nurse!*"

"I'll be there in a minute," I respond and rush off to help my co-worker lift and reposition their patient.

On the inside, I can feel tightness in my breathing, my shoulders elevated up to my ears, vibrations in my chest and sheer frustration with not having enough time or hands. Completely overwhelmed by the imbalance between what I've already done and what still needs to be done.

In our society of hustle, grind, and stress we are living in "fight or flight" a large portion of the time. Our sympathetic nervous system, part of our autonomic nervous system, is responsible for helping keep us safe, to escape danger, whether physical, emotional, or mental. When this system is activated, our resources are diverted to vital organs and muscles (the things that help us escape, think running) and we slip into survival mode. Adrenaline and cortisol are released, this is where that boost of energy comes from when you are scared or feel threatened—the energy that helps you run away. The same release (cortisol/adrenaline) happens when you ride a scary ride at the amusement park, which can be exhilarating and fun, but in short intervals. This response is meant to be short-lived. Hanging out in sympathetic mode for long periods of time can be damaging.

Living in an ongoing stimulation/activation of the sympathetic nervous system leads to chronic stress that can lead to disease and illness. Think high blood pressure, inflammation, anxiety and digestive issues, feelings of unfulfillment, and lack of motivation to name a few. This can affect our energy levels and lead to burnout and adrenal fatigue. Our sympathetic nervous system's job is to increase our heart rate and blood pressure so our body can respond to the danger it is in (or thinks that it's in).

Our parasympathetic nervous system, our "rest and digest" healing mode, helps us achieve and maintain homeostasis within the body. Our parasympathetic nervous system aids in maintaining a healthy balance physically and mentally. I have worked in a profession for over thirty years that has conditioned me to always push and push and then push more—*do, do, do*. Constantly racing the clock, racing time, and chasing life. An industry that encourages me to work more, rest less, and put myself last. As a perpetual "DO-er" and someone addicted to DOing, falling into and staying in this vicious cycle is easy and unhealthy.

It struck me recently how much of my life I have lived in "fight" mode. My sympathetic nervous system was completely in charge. It feels like clinging to an edge or hanging by a mere thread. This wasn't a conscious choice but rather the result of my internal and external environment. It became my default. Have you ever considered what side of your nervous system you are living in? Or how it is contributing to how you feel? Working as a nurse, especially in the ER, I live in this hyper-alert state constantly. This state *saves lives*! When there is a code or resuscitation situation, I mentally shut down, disengage from any present emotions, put my head down and GO! Hyper focused on the task at hand, my "running from the tiger" in health care. This state has completely drained me and continues to drain me. I spend my shift looking for, waiting for, and anticipating problems/emergencies. *All the time.*

I am hyper-vigilant of my environment because our safety can be at risk. I am hyper-vigilant about my patients and what is going on with them. I am hyper-vigilant about workload and the best way to tackle it most efficiently. I am hyper-vigilant all the time. All while knowing things could change in an instant, a moment, a literal heartbeat. Add in the constant noise of the environment around me, patient call bells going off, numerous people talking, patients yelling out, swearing, babies crying, IV alarms, cardiac monitors alarming, oxygen (sat) probes binging, and overhead pages—I can feel the vibration in my chest start to build. The effects of stress in my body, knowing every single one of my cells are absorbing this, and can the damn phone quit ringing for a minute! I feel like I might lose my mind but instead, I block out the sounds as best I can and shove those feelings way down deep, for another time (maybe), put my head down and keep on doing—there are eight more hours of my shift left.

7:00 am, dayshift starts, by 7:30 am I've had a report (that sometimes takes thirty minutes itself), I've been in to see two of my patients, taken both their vitals and charted them. I feel optimistic and hopeful for the shift ahead. Then 8:00 am hits and I've said, "Fuck!" more times than I care to count! Knowing the day has headed south real fast and I don't mean south where the beaches and margaritas are! Feeling overwhelmed and frustrated with the constant interruptions before I can even collect my thoughts for the day. I can *feel* the energy building in the department. It is becoming tense, chaotic, frantic, the air vibrating with the energy of every human in it. As my mental energy wanes my hyper-vigilance kicks in even more. An almost holding of my breath sensation at the base of my throat, my heart rate picking up speed as I try to avoid all the sensations, locking them away so as not to hinder my work or vomit them all over the trauma room floor.

A headache begins to intensify across my forehead along with the tension in my neck. I'm pretty sure the lack of water intake (I have had three sips) isn't helping and I haven't even finished the coffee I brought with me this morning! I've been at work for six and a half hours, the glass of water I had before leaving home eight hours ago isn't cutting it anymore, my mouth is dry, I can feel sweat rolling down my back, perspiration beads across my upper lip and I have sweat across my forehead under my mask and shield I've had on for six and a half hours.

I wonder to myself; can they see the sweat rolling down the side of my face? If only I could get a minute I could grab a few sips of water, but the patients keep coming.

People would not want to be in my head when I hear, "You guys are doing well." Um, *no we aren't*, we are anything but well, we are barely surviving right now! Paddling our arms hard to keep our heads above water trying to keep people alive. It's like running around slapping band-aids on a hemorrhage—it's the bare minimum. An IV here, an ECG there, here's a med, there's a med, everyone gets a med med. Just like Old MacDonald's farm, a quack quack here and a quack quack there. The patch phone goes off again for the fourth time in five minutes—we already have five EMS stretchers on offload delay lining the hallways. I swear if they would just stop coming, give us a little break maybe we could get ahead.

Imagine, you are a top spinning faster and faster, momentum and energy building, the energy inside of me trying to stay in control but threatening to spill out. This isn't the calibre of care I'd like to give. Could I have five minutes to do the procedure I need to get done and complete it calmly, not like my hair is on fire?

I have worked in this environment for over thirty years. This environment is not improving. It is only getting worse. Seeing a larger volume of patients, the acuity (how sick the patient is) is higher. "Shoulder season" is a period in which patient numbers are typically reduced, are in fact not. The ER is often full of admits with nowhere to go, a waiting room full of people to be seen and EMS on offload delay. There isn't more staff to handle the load, resources are not abundant, and the pay certainly hasn't increased. With the weight of responsibility nurses carry, work-load and lack of resources, you can start to imagine the inadequacies and potential for burnout. Nurses not only carry *their* workload, but that of other departments who are struggling with workloads and lack resources and staff as well. That work falls onto the nurses' shoulders (lab work, clerical duties and caring for admitted patients who can't be taken to the floors).

A Monday morning starts with a patient nearly tipping over the EMS stretcher, while still secured to it; yelling, screaming pro-fanities, out of control at 7:03 am.

I think silently to myself, (or I may have said it out loud), "I haven't had enough damn coffee for this yet!"

(Remember to breathe Peggy, I think).

OH NO, my sweet little elderly lady being investigated for diar-rhea needs changing again. . . C-diff—if you know, you know.

My temples start throbbing. I wish the volume in the depart-ment would settle down a decibel or two. . .and if one more person yells out *Nurse*, my head might explode!

Like a champagne bottle that was shaken, pressure waiting to explode when the cork pops. This is what it feels like inside my body.

This pressure builds as each hour passes.

I wonder. . . *am I going to lose it*? I wish I didn't pick up this shift. How many hours are left? I still have orders to check. How does this not get any better?

Life in the ER is chaos.

I push down all that I am feeling, bottle it all up, in hopes that somewhere down the road I can make space to 'deal with it'.

Commuting into every shift I silently ask myself, not *if* we will be short again but *how* short will we be today. Every shift I walk away from I feel a level of trauma embedded in my cells, stuck to my soul. A unique form of PTSD all on its own. The year 2021 has sent many nurses over the edge questioning their mental health and their profession. Where they were hanging on before, that rope has finally let go. Nurses have had it! The trauma experienced by nurses during this pandemic has not even been touched on. An entire book series in itself.

I always wanted to be a nurse, not sure exactly why (although as a people pleaser and doer, it's the perfect profession). I remember wanting to help others and thinking nursing was a reliable profession that paid well (stop laughing), as I know how ironic that is now. And bless my heart, never knowing 2020 was coming. I am *very* familiar with the fight or flight mode. Spending much of my life in this survival mode and now knowing more, how I felt/feel makes more sense. I can look back and see as a child who grew up in a home with a lot of turmoil, I was always in hyper-alert mode, always seeking to "keep the peace" or "not rock the boat," but instead do what was necessary to keep that peace—to settle the tumultuous boat. I can describe much of that period as walking on eggshells. There were good times and there was a lot of hypervigilance to what was going on around me, dissecting others' behaviours, moods, and body language. Waiting for the preverbal ball to drop.

Early into my teen years, I found myself speeding up life's milestones, finding myself in a stage of life prematurely—pregnant and scared at not quite fifteen years old. I hid this for several months, frightened someone would find out. I was hyper-alert about what I wore and how I looked and kept how I was feeling hidden away. As the news came to light some of my unspoken fears came to fruition, I heard whispers as I walked by. I was told I would not amount to much, I "wouldn't get far," that I'd "ruined" my life. My internal dialogue rose, "You want to fucking bet?"

The comments, the glares and stares I received, when support would have been better, fuelled my determination to prove them all wrong! This time in my life might have been where *doing* kicked into a supercharged mode and cemented into my DNA. I had a relentless desire to make a better life for myself, my baby and to prove everyone wrong. Every single one of them. However, that took a lot of DOing and zero BEing. I put my head down, built a solid wall around my heart, and hid my emotions spending the next number of years DOing, rinsing and repeating that behaviour. If you are there now or recently have been, do not let this experience define who you are. This experience will shape who you are meant to be and who you are becoming. **Do not let others' thoughts and opinions be the trajectory of your life. Don't write yourself off**. They cannot define your future, as much as they might try. No matter how strong their opinions or how loud they shout them—you are in control of your future.

My DOing behaviour is what propelled me through high school, nursing school and every continuing education course I ever took thereafter. Today, I thank every one of those people who doubted me, some of whom I have treated throughout my nursing career. Oh, the irony.

How can you tell your scale is completely out of balance? First, you're going to feel it, like inside your body *feel* it. I will share with you some of the feelings and behaviours I noticed on repeat.

I felt:

- Super exhausted all the time but kept doing all the things (you would never have known).
- Lack of motivation.
- Decrease in mood.
- Negative self-talk (the things I would say on repeat in my head about myself).
- Feeling like a failure when things I desired didn't go as planned.
- Feeling stuck.
- Guilt for thoughts and feelings.
- Jealousy of others.
- Burnt out.
- Wanting the fuck out—like there had to be something better/ easier way to make a living.

Behaviours I repeated:

- Wasting time.
- Lack of focus/clarity.
- Procrastination.
- Do another thing, do more, fill my time.
- Fill my days.
- Compare myself to others.
- Poor time management (see number one).
- Do more for others.
- Wander around with no idea where to start.
- Searching for outside validation (achievement, I know this well).

Things I have done in the last 18 months:

- Wrote a chapter in 2 collaborative books.
- Completed 200 hr meditation teacher training.
- Completed 200 hr Yoga teacher training.
- Spent 7 weeks at my daughter's helping her in another province with a newborn & almost 2-year-old.
- Completed 2 biz programs each being 12 and 14 weeks.
- Closed my dad's estate as executor.
- Launched my signature program.
- Podcast interviews.
- Hosted Zoom calls connecting with nurses.
- Welcomed 3 additions to the family.
- Guest speaker in groups.
- Numerous FB and Instagram lives.

- Ran an online retreat for nurses.
- Living life outside the ER and my family life—which is very busy.
- Working 12 hr day and night shifts in the ER.
- I host a book club.
- Spending hundreds of hours on my laptop working to start a business.

Just to name a few. I tell you this to show you the number of things I do that have contributed towards me moving away from BEing, even when I thought it was aligned! Here is the comedy in it all, my doing led to being! BEing encompasses DOing. Maintaining homeostasis in the mind, body and soul is key. The doing has changed however, because it has become very intentional. There came a time in my life and my career when it all caught up to me. I felt completely out of balance. It felt uncomfortable enough to stop, to evaluate and determine what was going on and why. I could not even explain the feeling. Like something was missing. My tank was drained, I was not taking intentional time to fill it. I was burning the candle at every end, in fact, my candle had wicks on every side and they were all on fire! I was a hot mess. I did more. Classic Peggy. It took a few more years to finally see how much I had been living in fight or flight mode and survival mode with a cortisol level running rampant.

I became tired of being tired and wanting more out of life (yes, even when my life was already great) I knew there was more. The more was being. The more was the mind, body, and soul connection. The more I discovered was *me*. And I didn't realize how much it was me until I was writing these words, in this chapter.

BEing encompasses DOing. Maintaining homeostasis in the mind, body and soul is key.

I accidentally fell into a journey where I learned more about myself, what I truly wanted and what matters most. What I had been looking for was a way to replace my nursing income so I could get the hell out of dodge. I was looking for an income without the restraints of geographical location. I wanted an abundant income where I dictated the rules because nursing is fucking hard—at least my type of nursing in the ER. So, what did I do? I invested in myself, again and again, and again. Initially investing in events and workshops, moved on to group programs and then on to private coaching or mentorship. And books, I love books!

I became *aware* of what was happening and the repetitive patterns I kept falling into.

How did I change this?

- Self-awareness was KEY!
- Determining my core values (HUGE).
- BOUNDARIES! (This is M-A-S-S-I-V-E).

- Perspective shifts (Life CHANGING).
- Self-care (CRUCIAL).
- Getting intentional with my days (VALUABLE).
- Breath (VITAL).

Awareness, if you don't know, you don't know, and therefore you cannot create change. And when you know, you can never unknow. So, get super clear on your core values and your priorities in life!

Suggested Exercise:

Core values are the standards you set for your life, your priorities. Grab a pen and take the next five minutes for you. Write down things that are super important to you that are priorities in your life. This could be health, family, integrity whatever those are to you, not anyone else. Go ahead I'll give you five. . . (did the jeopardy theme song just start playing in your head?)

Now, circle the five that are your highest priorities. TAH DAH! These are your core values! When you feel stuck making a decision, ask yourself, does this thing align with my core values? Does saying yes align with my values? There is your answer!

Side note: you can do this exercise over and over, your core values may shift throughout the seasons of your life. Think being single then becoming a spouse, priorities change. Think having babies, priorities change. It's a good exercise to come back to from time to time.

Diving into my core values brought an awareness like no other. I (finally) after considering it for years, changed my nursing position to a casual one, which allows me to control my schedule with flexibility. I now plan my work schedule around my life, instead of the other way around. This was a weight lifted off my shoulders, knowing I have a choice. It's like I have room to breathe. The flexibility is newfound freedom. Now, I fill out my calendar with the things I want to do, places I want to go *then* I add in my shifts.

I have learned to say no without explanation or guilt (for the most part). I say no to work more often than not. I was always the yes person, yes I'll fill that shift, yes I can come in—interrupting my life for work. When I feel I am struggling to say no (I still fall into old habits if I am not mindful), I pause, remind myself of my core values and do a check-in. Does my saying yes to this thing/this shift align with my core values and how I want to feel? If it is a, no it does not, then it's *hell no, thank you*! I have learned zero amount of money is worth my peace, my mental health, my sanity or ignoring my priorities (core values) or the standards I have set for myself. These are boundaries and boundaries are the highest form of self-respect anyone can have for themselves.

I learned about self-care (don't roll your eyes), there is a reason you hear the word often. This is crucial to a happy being, a fulfilled life, a feeling of peace and calm. I wish I could reinvent this word so people would not ignore it and think it's insignificant. *It is life-changing*! You can look up the phrase self-care anywhere, but my definition of self-care is *the intentional act and personal accountability of looking after one's self, mind, body and soul.* Self-care = tools that transform your life. I have a whole toolbox full of these that help me keep my tank full to maintain harmony.

This is work, every damn day.

Tools to slow the roll (morning routines, self-care, being intentional, yoga, meditation, getting outside, adventure whatever that means for you, breathing). Developing a morning routine changed my life. I now start my day in a quiet, calm, and intentional way. I dare you to try it. Really try it. I used to start the day tired when I woke up and hit the ground running, already feeling behind. I would run all day until I fell into bed at night, typically after 11:00 pm. I would lay down thinking of what I didn't get done, silently beating myself up about it all and how much more I had to do tomorrow! If I woke up during the night (often did) those thoughts would be swirling around in my head, as if I had never slept at all. When I woke in the morning, those thoughts were still swirling relentlessly. Rinse and repeat daily, I started the day like my hair was on fire and the day ran me from there. P.S. Those to-do lists you make are impossible for most humans.

Breathe.

Please, remember to breathe. Check-in, are your shoulders around your ears, breathing shallow breaths? Holding your breath? Breath is a hidden not used intentionally enough tool I never appreciated for years.

Of course, we all breathe (until we don't). I've learned my breath can help settle the crazy in my day and I can use it to decompress after my hectic shifts in the ER.

As a nurse, I should have known to do this all sooner, but remember the fight or flight mode, cortisol pumping through my body? Not only have I implemented yoga and meditation into my days, but I was determined to integrate them fully into my life and reap the benefits, and find stillness and space in my life. I went ahead (hello DOing) and completed my 200-hour meditation certification and 200-hour yoga teacher training. Here is where my awareness of the vagus nerve kicked in.

Meditation helps to activate the vagus nerve and engage the relaxation response connected with the parasympathetic nervous system. Breathing, heart rate, and gut health all influence and impact the vagus nerve which can send signals from body to brain and can trigger the relaxation response. Mind-body connection, are you starting to see it? it? These are tools for life, tools we carry with us every day, everywhere. Tools to completely reset the nervous system, the very system that is fried. When the sympathetic nervous system is overstimulated, we can influence our fight or flight response. We can do this by engaging the parasympathetic nervous system, through the vagus nerve. By slowing our breath and easing stress in and on our body, we can alert the brain that we are safe, creating mind, body connection. This super important, super supportive connection helps maintain homeostasis (balance) within our body. All vital to our well-being.

In the ER where I remind and tell people to breathe and too frequently fully support their breathing, I find myself forgetting to do it myself! When I take note of my breathing, I usually find it is shallow and all in my upper chest. I have to tell myself to take full, deep breaths, sometimes escaping to the bathroom to take them! If nothing else resonates from these words you've read, take this one thing away. The number of things you *do* does not equal your worth or your value, as a mom, a spouse, a friend, a nurse, an employee or as a human being! Deciding, thinking, striving, and doing is like a train gathering momentum, it can be hard to apply the brakes and it's exhausting. This took me a very long time, years to recognize.

Your worth is not, I repeat, is **not** based on the number of things you do.

Please know, I am not there yet (not even close). I've learned there is no final destination and I question my goodness daily, as I wonder how many "fucks" a day is too many. We have this great, big, beautiful journey we call life, and it is work. Every damn day. It has become the norm to think if you aren't doing something, hustling, that you are wasting time, unproductive and lazy (I believe society and social media contribute to this mentality). A reminder, DOing encompasses a multitude of tasks of varying complexities and takes a lot of mental energy. No human has an unlimited supply of that. Caring for yourself is the "magic" answer (trick) you are seeking for more energy.

We are meant to thrive, not merely survive, in this incredible life. It all starts with awareness and the conscious choice to create change. At the end of all of this, I will leave you with a mantra.

"I am worthy, not because of what I do but because of *who I am*."

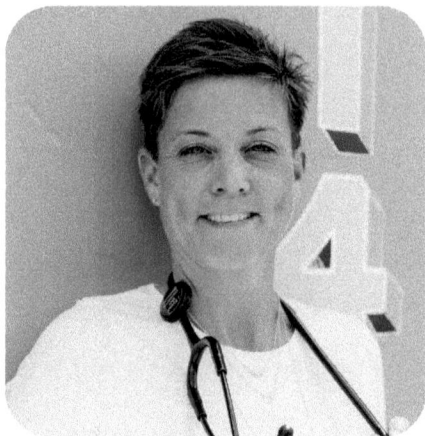

Peggy Birr

Peggy is known for her infectious energy, humour, love of adventure, travel, coffee, Malbec, reading and crystals. She loves the mountains, beaches and being outdoors, hiking, camping and soaking up mother nature's vibe. Peggy is very familiar with DOing and achieving. Peggy hit a period in life where she had to admit she was burned out, exhausted, knowing something had to change. While on a journey to create change and a positive impact in her life she realized what was missing, her BEing. She was living every day like it was an emergency, her nervous system fried, living in fight or flight all the time. Diving into the tools Peggy has and continues to use, she is finding more fulfilment, joy, energy and connection, mind, body and soul. Reconnecting with her BEing. These tools help keep her nervous system in check and find calm in the chaos of life and the ER. Peggy is a strong advocate and guide to help women move themselves UP their priority ladder and stay there—**guilt-free**. Peggy is a certified yoga and meditation teacher and ritual guide, whom you may find with a pocket full of crystals—insert the woo woo!

IG @peggybirr

FB @peggy.birr.79

Web peggybirr.com

John, the one that makes all I do possible, in so many ways. My wingman, my best friend, the one I can always count on. The one who walks beside me, especially on the hard days. Your support and encouragement mean more than I could express.

Jeff, Trista, Emily, our children. Hudson, Molly, Scarlett, and Leo, our grandbabies . . . the ones who are always watching. The ones who have taught me there is more love to give. My priorities, my Joy. I hope I lead by example, to be the best version of a human on this planet as possible.

Lastly, to my stronger self, I thank you. The one who continues, even on the hard days. I applaud you for your determination, perseverance, and resilience to just keep putting one foot in front of the other and for honouring yourself when you need to rest. Without you, these words would never be written.

CHAPTER FOUR

From Surviving to Thriving

Barb MacKay

My name is Barb, and I am a person in recovery. Childhood and adult sexual abuse, emotional and physical abuse, drug addiction and alcoholism, codependency, and an adult child of alcoholics, perfectionism, workaholism and prescription drug dependency. I am twenty-nine years clean and sober from alcohol and street drugs. I am a survivor, but most importantly, I am a thriver. I am a beautiful, strong, resilient woman. My hope is to inspire you to shake off the chains, to rise up and live your best life! This story is about my recovery from prescription drug dependence.

Functional Dyspepsia (FD) is what I navigate every day. By definition, "FD is a term for recurring signs and symptoms of ingestion that have no obvious cause."[1] But based on my health history, I can hypothesize a few probable causes. Here is a glimpse into what a typical day looks and feels like for me in this body.

I awake in the morning and feel acid in my stomach. Sometimes a lot,

1 Functional dyspepsia, https://www.mayoclinic.org/diseases-conditions/functional-dyspepsia/symptoms-causes/syc-20375709, Mayo Clinic, 2022

sometimes a little, either way, it feels gross and painful. Everything I ingest affects it. I feel panicky and scared. What if it overtakes me? But no, my body knows exactly what to do, I continually convince myself. I gingerly sip my tea after walking the dog and continue with my day, running errands, attending meetings, and doing laundry. I refuse to allow this feeling to overtake me. My stomach feels unsettled, but I refuse to throw up. The pain and random acid feelings pop and travel throughout my body. This sensation pulses in my abdomen and I am afraid to eat. In go the probiotics and collagen. Weird acidic reactions ensue, and my stomach feels empty. I try not to panic. The acid begins to build again. Now what? I continue with my day and try not to think about it. I look forward to bedtime. How will it feel laying in bed? Hopefully not a torture chamber like some nights. I begin to feel clammy and hungry again. I float through my day always worrying about the acid. It's relentless torture. It begins to rise and fall throughout my esophagus, flowing from my armpits to my stomach, incessantly. It's disgusting. I am so nervous and afraid. I wait, I write, I focus on more chores, and I drink water. Up and down the acid goes. It seems to be building and is very painful. I continue with my day. More walking with my dog. Finding more distractions. The acid continues to burn slowly into my stomach. Sometimes waves of it on my sides. Constantly building in my stomach. More pain. I have another cup of tea in the afternoon. Tea seems to cause the acid to increase, but then slowly dissipate afterwards. My day continues and this feeling returns. Rising and falling acid throughout my cells. My stomach begins to spasm. Stay with it. Walk. Drink more water. Feel the up and down of the food, the acid. It's painful. Drink lots of water and wait for it to subside. Time to take my night meds. Have some soup with toast. Acid rushes in. Feels tight, waiting for it to digest. Extremely painful and within forty-five minutes I feel the acid building again. I eat some yogurt. Same thing. Building. So painful, and it's only 7:00 pm! A long way out from bedtime. A bit more water. Down. Then up. Incessant. All day, every day. My coping strategies are varied. I try to ignore these extremely uncomfortable feelings in my torso, but it's difficult. I pretend they are something other than what they are. I rationalize them as warm and fuzzy and imagine I am safe and secure. It's horrible but I go on. I'm hoping by sharing this I will be relieved of all these feelings. They are getting less and less as I write.

This is a typical day of living inside my body. It is a neurological, physical, and emotional experience. As my body is listening to my brain, where the simple yet terrifying act of eating and drinking is so painful, I am stuck in a loop. How will my brain figure this out? How will my body figure this out? My nervous system is in overdrive and it's difficult for my brain to keep up with what is going on in my body. Consequently, I am not sleeping well and searching for ways to feel better so I can rest. Extreme tightness in my chest consumes my body. How could anyone sleep feeling this way? Never underestimate the power of anxiety, it started with this, my brain is struggling and my body is tired. Our brain's job is ultimately to protect us from pain, which means it anticipates where it thinks pain is going to be, long before we eat or move. Am I ever going to sleep? How can I cope when I can't sleep, then awake for hours in the night, drinking water, it is unrelenting, even breathing brings feelings, and I honestly don't want to go there but I know I have to. I feel like I am faking it all the time, I just want to be normal, but I don't even know what normal is anymore. It feels like hell inside my body, and I want to break this loop. I am scared to eat so I don't. I wait for my body to catch up. I am not staying in the present and I have difficulty with memory and anxiety. I have been in a panic attack for four years.

In March 2006, I hurt myself at work while lifting an 18L water bottle onto the cooler injuring my lower back. This began my journey into physical dependency with prescription medication. At first, I was prescribed medications for pain, anxiety, and depression. This was the beginning of a three-year battle with the Workers Compensation Board (WCB) to obtain disability benefits. During this time, I was required to take certain medications as prescribed by their doctors, to see one of their psychiatrists, and to attend intense physiotherapy for four to six hours per day in their rehab facility. I was required to stay away from my home for months and lived in a hotel alone, driving to and from the hotel to the facility each day. Looking back, I know this was not the best practice and it shouldn't have happened this way.

The following year I was in a car accident that totalled my vehicle. This was caused by the strong pain medication I was required to take. Studies have shown antipsychotics, benzodiazepines, and high-potency opioids increase crash risks by up to 35%. Very disturbing statistics. Luckily, no one was injured other than me. I was then diagnosed with whiplash, a shoulder injury, and my back pain increased. The pain medication was changed to a stronger one and I was prescribed additional medications for nerve pain and back spasms. I was living in a semi-comatose state.

In 2008, I was in yet another car accident, again totalling my vehicle without hurting anyone else, thank goodness! My back, shoulder and neck pain worsened. In addition to this, my marriage was suffering as my husband left home to pursue a lucrative position in the oil sands. I was left with no income and began seeing a therapist to help me come to terms with losing my career. My thirty-year career as an accountant/bookkeeper, along with my achievements now seemed insignificant. I was devastated.

After the second accident, I decided to check myself into a detox facility to withdraw from the heavy pain medication. After ten days, I went home to recover. I had horrible withdrawal symptoms including rage, suicidal ideation, incessant pain, nausea, sweating, chills, diarrhea, stomach cramps and muscle aches. This lasted a few months but after six months I began to feel a lot better. That being said, I still had to take all medications required by the WCB. I had to have my prescription filled for the pain medications even though I didn't ingest them. I was switched to other medications and my anti-anxiety medication increased. I worked with an advocate to obtain my WCB Disability and CPP Disability and finally obtained this income.

My husband was still away at work and I had responsibilities at our country acreage, including maintenance of the grounds, overseeing extensive renovations to our home, and caring for up to ten dogs we were raising and breeding. I was mostly alone and when my husband came home on his time off, he took over these responsibilities. One winter night while out feeding the dogs I slipped on the ice and cracked the back of my head. Now, I had a concussion on top of it all.

During this stressful period, I had a severe outbreak of psoriasis. My scalp, face, hands, and neck were covered. I saw a dermatologist and was prescribed four different types of hydrocortisone, one for each area. A shampoo for the scalp and three different kinds of cream. Today it only occurs when I am stressed and at the change of seasons and is quite manageable with one cream.

In 2010, I was hospitalized because the depression and anxiety had left me in an unbearable state. During this brief hospital stay in a psychiatric ward, my anti-anxiety dosage was doubled. I was attacked by another patient, punched repeatedly on the head and face, and had a laceration under my eye from my glasses hitting my face. My glasses were broken. The hospital agreed to pay for new glasses but refused to take any responsibility for the incident. I was encouraged to leave the hospital and go home and rest. Upon leaving, I reverted to my previous dosage of anti-anxiety medication.

In 2015, my husband and I decided to spend part of the winter in Arizona. When I attended my physician's office, I was given prescriptions for three months. My doctor suggested I switch my medication for my depression. This made things much worse. I did however switch the antidepressant. It took me one whole year of horrid symptoms to get on and then off this nasty drug. Our holiday was ruined—I spent most of it in bed. Naturally, my husband and family were very concerned and upset.

When I returned home my doctor prescribed medication for sleep. I was like a zombie, practically in a coma. My life was a living hell. I barely made it from the bed to the couch, sleeping eighteen hours a day. My husband was beyond frustrated. I was confused and I became the patient and him, my caregiver. He had retired and was home 24/7. This continued until 2017. I could not participate in daily life. My anxiety was extreme. I did not know it at the time, but I had been experiencing inter-dose withdrawal from the anti-anxiety medication.

In March 2017, my eldest son died from a drug overdose. I was devastated. We travelled to Vancouver to take care of the funeral arrangements. We had to wait two weeks for the coroner to release his body at the funeral home. He had to go through testing for fentanyl poisoning as this was amid the Overdose Crisis. He had been mostly clean and sober for the previous two years. He had suffered for many years with mental health and addiction issues and took many of the same medications I was prescribed. We spoke on the phone daily. He was starting a new job. It was very exciting. One thing he said to me that began my journey to wellness that I will never forget was, "You have to get up and fight, mom." He decided to use drugs one last time, and tragically it was the last day of his life.

My younger son was also in recovery from drug addiction. I am proud and happy to say that he is ten years living clean and sober, has an amazing job, a girlfriend, and a beautiful daughter. He has healthy hobbies and pursuits including hiking and camping as well as being an accomplished photographer.

I began seeing a grief counsellor to deal with the loss of my eldest son and it became apparent to her the medication and my inconsolable grief would have to be dealt with. My marriage was unhealthy, and I needed to make some major changes. In September 2017, I left the marriage and moved home to British Columbia. I had been in contact with an old friend from forty years before and he offered me a safe place with no conditions. I left in the middle of the night with a tote bag and caught a plane.

By now I was in a constant panic attack and could not think straight. Once I moved back to B.C. I began to formulate a plan to get off as many medications as possible. I had started with all the pain medications, now it was time to tackle the benzodiazepines. In April of 2018, I entered a detox facility and stopped all of these medications cold turkey. This was the beginning of a new hell on earth. I was to be in a protracted withdrawal state for the next four years. This was difficult and dangerous. I could have a seizure and die. At times I wished for this. I was in a constant state of panic. I was hypersensitive to sound, touch, light, smell, and taste. I had OCD and PTSD. I experienced tremors and akathisia. Abnormal body sensations which were very disturbing and painful, auditory, visual, and tactile hallucinations.

Depersonalization and derealization were my daily companions. I was agoraphobic and afraid of everything both inside my home and out. I had constant intrusive thoughts and active suicidal ideation. I thought about suicide and researched ways to do it daily. I had severe gastrointestinal symptoms including diarrhea and pain in my gut and feelings of weird pressure and the feeling of food being stuck in my body. I lost weight—over forty pounds, and I had insomnia. I was irritable and felt a lot of rage. My thoughts were very aggressive, mostly towards myself. I experienced confusion and dizziness. I had cognitive difficulties and memory problems. I felt constant nausea but could not throw up. I had heart pain and palpitations. I had a constant headache and dry mouth, fatigue, muscle pain and weakness. I experienced night sweats and nightmares while awake. I had paranoia and thought others were reading my thoughts. It was a traumatic brain injury. I had windows and waves. Waves were the roughest of times and I had glimpses of windows of sanity and peace. Mostly waves for a long time.

In September 2018, I travelled to Vancouver to see a doctor at the University of British Columbia that had agreed to help me taper off the rest of the medications. I moved into a small basement apartment near my family. I am so grateful for their love and support during this turbulent time. I travelled weekly to see this doctor by bus and Skytrain, a four-hour return trip. My anxiety, agoraphobia and akathisia were so severe that I had a supportive friend text to talk me through it. I also began seeing a therapist and practiced focusing, tapping and other modalities in an attempt to deal with these issues.

As a recovering alcoholic, I attended 12 Step meetings several times per week and practiced grocery shopping and walking alone in the city. I socialized with my family and helped with housework and childcare as I was able. I made a few new friends and enjoyed our gatherings for coffee and lunch. My active suicidal ideation was the most challenging. I wanted to die every day for three years and researched ways to do it. I never attempted any of them but fantasized about it constantly. I got through one minute at a time. I could not sleep and spent my nights writhing in my pain and agony and watching copious amounts of serial television. I paced, I chanted, I prayed, and I shook inside and out. I cried. I was hospitalized briefly a few times and given antipsychotic medications for my symptoms and inability to sleep. I was becoming a burden to my family. I developed severe gastrointestinal issues and was prescribed proton pump inhibitors for acid reflux in December 2019.

This coincided with my withdrawal from the antipsychotic medication. I did not know what was going on with my body. The PPIs seemed to make things worse. My doctor there had prescribed a non-addictive medication for my anxiety. I had constant diarrhea and gut pain with weird sensations all over my body. Painful and concerning. My doctor increased my antidepressant to three times my original dose. I had all kinds of tests and exams for my digestive issues. I was given a GI scope and a colonoscopy. Nothing turned up and I was at my wit's end.

Finally, in March 2020, I returned to my companion's home in the interior. Two weeks later he was diagnosed with cancer and given six months to live. Again, more devastation was felt and now he needed my support. I began driving which I had not done for two and a half years. I took him to his chemotherapy and radiation treatments. It was very frightening. I believe I had PTSD due to my previous car accidents and everything that occurred and everything that was still occurring. I was no longer suicidal by the summer of 2020. I supported him and loved him up until his passing in November 2020. During that time there were restrictions due to the covid epidemic. We talked, we laughed, we loved, we did jigsaw puzzles and watched many movies. He was my soulmate.

During that time, I was prescribed every PPI possible and I was taking these multiple times a day, not eating, but drinking large amounts of water. I had another GI scope and colonoscopy and again no adverse results. After my soulmate passed, I was hospitalized. It was there it was suggested I had a Functional Neurological Disorder. I researched this and attempted to see a specialist on this in Victoria, B.C. I was

I am determined to keep fighting and live my best life, doing it one day at a time, sometimes one hour at a time.

not successful, and the program is now closed. I believe the residual of all the medications and my protracted withdrawal are the culprits. These digestive issues and weird and painful feelings are getting less daily but still occurring. The GABA receptors in my gut are still healing.

I am determined to keep fighting and live my best life, doing it one day at a time, sometimes one hour at a time. I am praying soon I will be *normal* and can live free of the residual damage I struggle with, especially the FND. It's a constant battle, but I soldier on. My mental health is good, and I cherish my freedom from all the meds, building a good life for myself and have recently met a special person. We spend time together walking our dogs and getting away on jaunts to the city. We are planning a trip to Mexico this winter. I never would have believed I would have the life I do today. It has been a hard-fought battle and I will continue to fight for my freedom from the chains of physical dependence on prescription medication.

In telling my story, and hopefully helping others, I am trusting my healing will be complete and I can get on with my new life. I am off all prescription medications except for hormone replacement therapy and a low-dose antidepressant which I am currently tapering. I have a beautiful apartment in a small town and a beagle puppy, living alone and making new friends. I feel mostly happy, joyous, and free. I believe myself to be 99.9% healed. The gastro issues are getting lighter and lighter as I write this story and as the days go by. My hope is they will disappear as all these thoughts and feelings reach the light of day. Out of me and onto the paper. I attended a 12-Step Program and recently had an amazing six-week trip to Vancouver Island and the Lower Mainland to visit friends and family. Gratitude rises in my heart daily. I made it and you can too. In my son's words,

"Get up and fight warriors. For your sanity, for a good life and a happy ever after."

It can be done, and I am living proof!

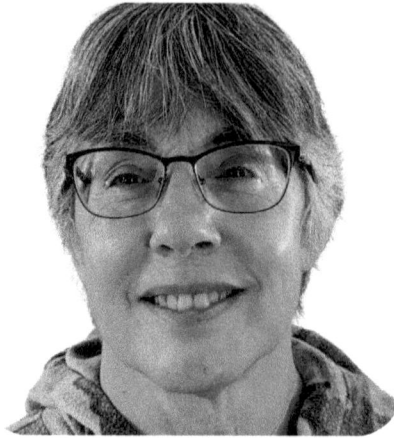

Barb MacKay

Barb MacKay is a person in recovery living in the Cariboo region of B.C. She lives with her dog Gypsy and is enjoying life to the fullest. She is mostly happy, joyous and free. Born and raised on Haida Gwaii (Queen Charlotte Islands) she has lived in many places including Nova Scotia and all over British Columbia. She is a survivor and a thriver. She helps others where she can and attends 12-Step meetings weekly. She volunteers with a local community group and spends her time with friends and family. She is currently seeing a new friend and is enjoying time with him and his dog. She is outgoing and healthy.

IG @msbarbaradhl | FB @barb.mackay.56

I would like to thank the following people for their part in loving and supporting me on my journey. My sons Ian and Elton, may he Rest In Peace, Mom and Dad, Sharon and Ron, my sister Susan and her husband Marty, my nieces Jill, Jenna and Jessi and their families, my best friend Linda, my friend Marlene, Dr. James M. Wright of UBC, my friend Wes, may he rest in peace, my friends in the 12-Step community, and my dog Gypsy. Also my new friend Barry and his dog, Benny. I could not have done this without you.

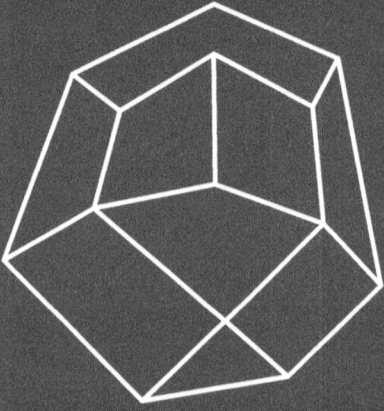

CHAPTER FIVE

Breast Cancer: A Journey of Self Discovery and Healing

Jillian Price

My name is Jillian Price, and I am a breast cancer survivor. I never thought I would be saying that, especially at age forty-three. I was diagnosed right after my fortieth birthday. I discovered a small bump very close to the surface of my skin on my right breast just above my nipple. I didn't do anything about it for about a month and then showed it to my husband. We both agreed better to be on the safe side and get it checked. I made an appointment with my family doctor who upon examination thought it felt like a cyst. Neither of us was overly concerned but both agreed I should get a mammogram just to be sure. About a month later, there I was at the Breast Cancer Clinic, getting my very first mammogram and not feeling that worried. Why should I be? I was too young to get cancer, right?

It's important to note that I wasn't feeling sick at all. I was living a pretty healthy lifestyle. I had been going to the gym regularly for over a year. I was in the best shape of my life upon diagnosis. I had been a smoker on and off since high school; more off than on in my later years once I got married and started having kids. I probably didn't have the best diet, but it wasn't horrible. I had no serious chronic illnesses, never broken a bone, wasn't on any medications and I thought my mental health was solid.

At my first mammogram appointment, I had no idea what a normal procedure was. Now that I have been through this procedure several times, I noticed they took a lot more images than they normally do. When they were finished, I was told I would have to come back for a contrast mammogram and biopsy. Now the hairs on the back of my neck began to tingle and I began to wonder, should I be worried? I returned about a week later and they took me into a different room to meet with a nurse navigator. She explained what procedures I would be getting done. That's when the real worry started to set in. Why all this, if it was only a cyst?

Waiting for the results of the biopsy was torture. I did my best to stay busy and focus on other things but looking back, I'd say waiting for results at many different points in my treatment was the worst part of it all. Once you know what you are working with and what needs to be done, then it's all about making decisions. But the weeks of tests and consultations followed by periods of waiting are pure torture. And in the beginning, there is a lot of waiting and uncertainty.

I remember the moment vividly. I was given the news; they had found cancer. I was out of town at a business meeting with a group of my colleagues. We had decided to meet for lunch before a long afternoon of meetings. I was in the parking lot at the restaurant when my phone rang. My family doctor was the one to give me this life-changing news—she was just as shocked as I was. I ended the call abruptly and sat in my car feeling completely shell-shocked. I couldn't even believe what I had just heard. I couldn't process it. I had just received the worst news of my life, alone, and nowhere near home. Not knowing what else to do, I went on auto-pilot and walked into the restaurant and tried to get through the day, but I couldn't eat anything, sitting in silence. My colleagues asked me if I was okay, and I lied saying I wasn't feeling well. I tried to get through the meetings until finally realizing I had to get home.

My official diagnosis was estrogen receptor-positive (ER-positive) invasive mammary carcinoma. ER-positive breast cancer is the most common type of breast cancer in women. Interestingly, the original small bump that we suspected was a cyst had mysteriously just disappeared on its own. It was like my body put it there and took it away just as quickly. Like it was a signal to get my attention and once it did, it was gone. I was told this cancer was probably growing inside my body for the last three to five years and I likely wouldn't have felt the lump on my own for quite some time given the location deep in my breast behind my nipple.

The appointments with oncologists happened fast once I was officially diagnosed. During those medical appointments, I felt completely numb. I don't think I spoke two words in those initial appointments. I just sat there and listened to them talk about terrifying things like the grade and stage of my tumour, survival rates, and the chance of recurrence. Not to mention the long list of potential procedures and treatments I would have to endure like mastectomy, chemotherapy, and radiation followed by at least five years of taking the oral hormone therapy drug Tamoxifen. Each time I would leave the hospital in a completely comatose state. I couldn't wrap my head around how this could happen to me. I think I had this naive notion when people get cancer, they know something is wrong because they feel sick, but that's not how it works at all, or at least not in my case. I wasn't sick! What had I done wrong in my life to get cancer so young? I immediately went on a search to figure out how I got here. I would typically go to books, science, and accredited medical websites to get my answers, but something told me the answers I was looking for wouldn't be found in those resources. I knew I needed to find the unconventional answers, the hidden answers, the truth.

Search for the cause. The reason this is happening.

I turned to alternative medicine. I had started my journey into alternative medicine a few years before I was diagnosed when I had a significant change in my body. In retrospect, I believe this was the beginning of my body trying to tell me something was wrong. About two years prior, my body started changing. It started to tell me something was wrong but not in the way I thought it would when your body is fighting cancer. I began to experience what I believe were symptoms of hormonal imbalance. My face began to break out and not the normal breakouts I was used to my whole life. As an adult, I've never had clear skin, but this was different! I began to get cystic acne. It was sore and relentless and crushing to my confidence. My career requires me to be in front of people all the time and all I wanted to do was hide until it was over. I started with the normal things by going to see my family doctor who prescribed several topical treatments, none of which I wanted to use. My body was telling me, this isn't going to work. *Search for the cause. The reason this is happening.* During that time, I also felt different. My moods were unstable, and I felt emotional all the time. I felt foggy, not like myself. I turned to naturopathy for some answers and with my naturopath, we worked on several things such as diet changes, liver detox and hormonal balancing with supplements. Things did get better. At this point, I certainly wasn't thinking I felt off because I had an estrogen-hungry tumour growing inside my body.

This previous experience with naturopathy sent me on a hunt to find as much information as possible that the medical oncologists weren't telling me. Not because they didn't care but because it wasn't how they were trained to treat cancer. What I was looking for couldn't be found in medical textbooks, but I believed I could help myself and my body fight this foreign thing trying to take over it. So began my search to understand how I ended up here in the first place. What was my body lacking, needing, or dealing with that was making it break down? I also realized I was going to have to do something I had never really done before in my life. I was going to have to talk to people and share my story with others if I wanted them to do the same. This was incredibly difficult for me to do as anyone who knows me well knows I'm a woman who was pretty guarded with her personal life and kept her emotions to herself; certainly not the kind of girl who sought out a friend to unload all her troubles. Not much girl talk happening over here! If I had something going on, I worked it out in my head. I talked myself through it. It was almost like I felt talking about it would make me feel worse—strange, but true. This was the first time in my life I actively went looking for advice and for people to talk to. I wanted to talk to anyone and everyone willing. I wanted to hear all their stories.

Western medicine focuses on treating the disease, but the root cause is rarely discussed. My oncologists focused on how to remove cancer from my body. My feelings were: if I never know why my body couldn't fight off the cancer cells in the first place, how do I know I won't end up here again? I wanted to do everything I could to stop the pattern of behaviours contributing to the growth of cancer cells. I wanted to eliminate the triggers, a healthy body that wasn't compromised. I saw my cancer treatments as band-aids or fixes but they didn't guarantee I wouldn't fall into the same pattern. I wanted to be proactive, not reactive, eliminating everything from my life that was increasing my chances of cancer coming back.

One of the best things I did was to immediately find a GP that specializes in women's health and breast cancer. I heard about this doctor from another breast cancer survivor who recommended her. She has a great website with amazing resources at faceitbreastcancer.com. This was a pivotal moment in my journey. After seeing her for an initial consultation, I knew I was in the right place and things were going to be okay. Finally, someone was asking the right questions. She did a thorough case history so we could investigate what could have contributed to my diagnosis at such a young age. She shared with me that in her practice she had seen a common theme of a traumatic event or stressful time in these women's lives a few years before getting sick. She understood the importance of treating this disease holistically and I was so grateful for this.

The more people I spoke to and the more research I did, the more this common theme of emotional trauma began to appear. I came across a book called, Heal Breast Cancer Naturally: 7 Essential Steps to Beating Breast Cancer, written by Dr. Véronique Desaulniers. She too had gone on a search of the, *why me?* A question that lingered in my thoughts. She had been living a healthy lifestyle by all accounts and was diagnosed not once but twice with breast cancer. I highly recommend this book if you are looking for information about alternative preventative medicine. I learned so much but what resonated the most with me was something she outlined in the book, *a profile of the type of women getting breast cancer.* It is referred to as the "cancer personality." Essentially, it is a list of personality traits that can act as emotional triggers causing stress in the body and initiating the development of cancer cells. Many of these traits involve suppressed toxic emotions, an absence of healthy ways to release stress, taking on other people's burdens and putting their own feelings last. These women are highly motivated, hard-working, responsible, and successful but it all comes at a price. To the outside world, these women would be described as bad-ass, put-together, strong, and confident. But on the inside, thoughts of doubt, fear, anxiety, and pain exist. They are hurting. This resonated with me on so many levels.

Once I took a deep dive into my psyche, the journey this led me on was one of true self-discovery in a way I had never done before. I peeled away all the layers and reached the core of what I believed was making me sick. The hidden traumas of my life; the pain, the resentment I had been keeping, childhood trauma, marital trauma, and childbearing trauma. I had years of repressed feelings I was holding on to and didn't even know it. I have never been one to dwell on things and move on pretty quickly from negative events, emotions, and feelings. To others, that seemed like a strength but now I understand this was my coping mechanism. I never allowed myself to feel the emotions, to let them pass through my body and release them. Instead, I didn't allow myself to feel any of it. It was almost like I became emotionless. I would later realize the way I had been living my life was cowardly. I accepted what people did to me. If they hurt me, I forgave them and let it go so I could move on. But it was more because I was so scared of change. I realized I am scared of change! I was scared to be seen as a failure, so I made it work. I am scared of failure! I realize now I was living in fear. I was letting fear control my life. Our bodies hold these negative feelings and thoughts and manifest them in many ways. Maybe it's an aching back or sore neck. Maybe it presents as headaches or trouble sleeping. All of this needs to be examined and healed. I now understand true strength comes when we face our fears, anxieties, and emotions.

My ability to stay focused, driven, and overcome obstacles made me known as the strong one. This is and should be, a compliment but when you are told this enough times, you start to adopt this belief and place an expectation on yourself that you are not allowed to be weak, vulnerable or say out loud, "I'm not okay, I don't think I can handle this, I need help." The expectation that you can handle it doesn't allow room for any other response. That is how it started to feel for me. People expected I would be strong, so I had to be. I felt like my worth was tied to my achievements. I didn't feel like people loved me for who I was but more for what I had achieved in life. The journey I was on made me realize just how loved I really was. I remember clearly the 'ah-ha' moment of recognizing I was incredibly loved by the number of people who showed up to support me. I also realized by not letting people in or asking for help, I felt very alone a lot of the time. Once I allowed myself to let people in and accept their help, those feelings disappeared.

I was incredibly lucky to have an amazing network of women who showed up! Some of these women I was not especially close to, but they had been touched by cancer in their own lives. Some were strangers to me before this but had a story to share and came out to support me through mine. I will be forever grateful to these women. I was so deeply touched by every act, big or small. To thank them and celebrate my girl tribe, I invited this group of ladies to a Sunday brunch after I completed all my treatments. I wanted them to meet each other as this was a beautiful collision of my worlds; work friends, family members, close friends, dance mom friends, etc. I wanted them to feel the power in our collective stories only we as women can tell. Visually, I realized I was never alone for one day in this journey because I had all of them. I don't find it easy to express my feelings verbally, especially when the topic is an emotional one, so I wrote each one of them a heartfelt and personalized thank you and read each one out to the group during brunch. I still cried my eyes out reading it, but I needed the words to come out and preparing written speeches made this possible. Looking back, I am so happy I did it that way. It was healing for me to write those words and the love and energy in the room were amazing.

One huge takeaway from this entire experience was the true power of women and their strength. We have heard this many times but when it is revealed to you in all its beauty it really is something. Surround yourself with these women. Yes, you have men that will support you; your spouse, father, brother, friends, but your fellow girl tribe truly understands, relates, and can empathize with your experience. A part of my body is physically gone; essentially my right breast was skinned of all its tissue. This is a sexual part of the body, tied to desire, romance, sex, femininity, attractiveness, body image and of course, motherhood. The breast is complex in terms of what it represents so losing one is just as complex. You have thoughts like, *will I still feel pretty, attractive, sexy, feminine? Will I feel like a whole person, like a whole woman?* Only another woman can truly understand that.

Allowing myself to feel emotions and express them is a work in progress for me. But one thing I changed right away because of this experience was to tell people how I feel about them now. Connections in my life matter so much more to me now. I make time to connect with the people in my life who bring me joy. I tell people often I love them or if they have touched me in some way, I make sure they know it. Make time to connect with people, nature, artistry, or anything that feeds your soul and brings you happiness. For me, dancing brings me the purest form of joy, so I make it a point to include at least a few minutes of dancing into every single day of my life. I'm also more open with others now. I talk about the imperfections of my imperfect life. Before I would hold my cards close. This keeps me in touch with my emotions and my soul.

One of the reasons I chose to be part of this book was to push myself out of my comfort zone and continue to release my emotions positively. I did this for my daughter also whom I see so much of myself in. She too holds her cards close and finds it difficult to express herself. I see the pattern and of course, this worries me. If I can face my fears and be vulnerable and let her know it's okay to make mistakes, fall down, be imperfect and ask for help, maybe I can set her on a better path than mine. I hope she will be proud of this and learn a few things about her mother and maybe herself along the way.

Looking back, this whole journey has taught me to chill the fuck out! Things don't have to be perfect; my kids don't have to be, I don't have to be. I have less patience for people treating me poorly, I care less about what others think of me, and I don't have to be doing more to feel like I'm growing. I want to do things that matter now. I want to spend my time with people I truly like, people who can teach me things, people who want to be better too—spiritually not superficially. Research shows stress is a risk factor for breast cancer and we all have stress but it's what you do with the stress that matters. We need outlets to release. The gym, yoga, meditation, counselling, anything that heals the soul. Stress suppresses your immune system, and a suppressed immune system is the window of opportunity for cancer to grow in your body. **It is the fuel.**

I felt the best emotional health I ever had during those two years fighting cancer, imagine that! It was the wake-up call I needed to find more inner peace. During this process, I felt more grounded and calm within myself than I ever had. It made me reexamine everything in my life. When bad things happen, you can choose to be bitter about it or be better. I chose the latter. I want to leave you with a list of some of the changes I made as a result of my diagnosis. I believe these, along with traditional medical treatments saved my life and changed it for the better. This was not a death sentence, but rather a second chance at living a healthier happier life. I am in control of my happiness now.

1. Talk to people who have gone through it. This was the best thing I did. I learned so much from other people's stories. The *most important thing* came from one of those conversations with a stranger who was brave enough to share her story. She told me about the Oncotype DX test, and I am forever grateful to her.

2. Inquire about the Oncotype DX test. It changed everything for me. This test identifies who will and will not benefit from adjuvant chemotherapy, the magnitude of benefit if any, and the risk of recurrence. My results showed the benefit was so minimal that it was not worth putting my body through the short and long-term effects of chemo. This completely changed the course of my treatment. Without these results, I would have gone through 4-6 rounds of chemotherapy. Instead, my doctors agreed it was not beneficial and mastectomy plus radiation and Tamoxifen was enough. Talk about a game-changer!

3. If you do have to do radiation, take good care of your skin. I used a cream called, My Girls, and it protected my skin from burning or scarring. Visit faceitbreastcancer.com for more information on this product.

4. If you don't feel supported by your doctors, then change doctors! This is something I would normally never do but after recognizing this personality trait of never wanting to rock the boat was detrimental to me and my health, I did do this not once but twice, during the course of my treatment.

5. Track everything. Bring a notebook with you to every appointment and record everything because chances are you won't remember it all.

6. Bring someone to every appointment. Just do it! You will need a second set of ears. Trust me.

7. Do your own research from accredited sources. Don't only rely on what your doctors tell you. If you feel like there are gaps or your gut is telling you something doesn't feel right, seek answers from other sources.

8. Explore alternative medicine. For me, this included naturopathy, energy therapy, reiki, meditation, supplements, blood analysis, intermittent fasting, and switching to a keto diet.

9. Consider purchasing an infrared sauna. Sunlighten is the company I purchased mine from and it is very reputable. This will help with the release of toxins from your body which is extremely important for cancer prevention.

10. If you are offered genetic testing, I recommend you do it. I learned I do have a genetic mutation which does put me in a higher risk category for breast and colon cancer.

11. Ozone therapy. This increases the amount of oxygen in your body and can help reduce the clogging of blood cells, detoxify the liver,

decrease uric acid in the body, improve circulation and oxygen supply, kill viruses, bacteria, and fungus, and improve the activity of the white blood cells. Clinical studies support the use of ozone therapy as an adjuvant during cancer treatment.

12. Work through past trauma with the goal of letting go of all that negativity. Practice gratitude. This one I'm still working on, but it is the greatest gift cancer has given me. Yes, getting sick can be a gift. It gave me a different perspective on life and for this I am grateful.

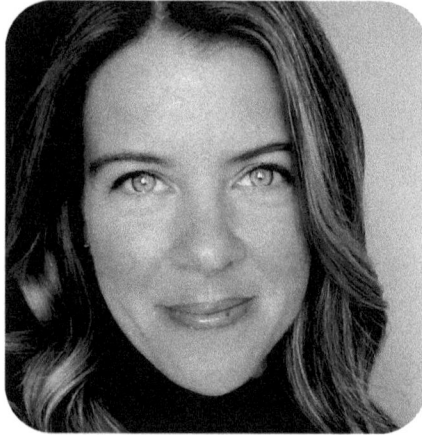

Jillian Price

Jillian Price lives in London, Ontario, Canada, and is a wife, mother of two, and senior executive working for a large national company in the field of Audiology. She has spent most of her life immersed in education, first as a student herself earning degrees in Psychology and Communication Sciences and Disorders from Western University, and later as an instructor teaching students and mentoring young graduates entering the profession of Audiology. She is passionate about education and sharing her knowledge with others. In her free time, Jillian finds joy in simple things. An impromptu kitchen dance party, watching movies, intimate gatherings with close friends, and spending time with her family are her favourite pastimes.

IG @jillprice_25

This chapter is dedicated to every woman, past, present, and future touched by breast cancer. May we continue to share our stories and show up for each other.

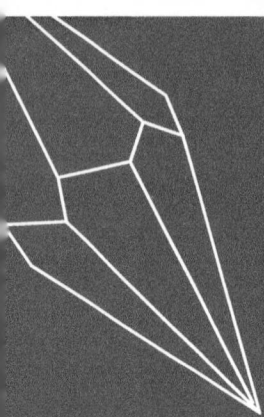

CHAPTER SIX

Burning It All Down

Jeanette Lucero

If the younger version of me would have had a glimpse into the forty-two-year-old me; no need for validation from men, not living for, "how my body looks," and no business or "job," she would have felt completely defeated as if she was going to be a failure in life. Yet, the stillness and security I now sit with and am blessed with every day at forty-two years young is the freedom I had searched for most of my life is indescribable to put into words.

Living in these constructs as a woman thinking women should look like "this" or "act like this" made me feel imprisoned in my body for a good part of thirty years. Yet during this time, I had been operating asleep, unaware, and unconscious as to how bad it was and had become. I was suffering as an asleep wounded woman eventually reaching a point of destruction and suicidal thoughts.

I remember being told as a little girl "a girl doesn't sit like that" or "that's not lady-like" so often I felt I must have been a failure at being a girl. Either that or I wasn't supposed to be a girl. So, who was I? I had a very muscular frame, excelled in gymnastics (which made me carry an even more muscular frame), I was raised by a very "tomboyish" mother, and most of all I lived with three brothers and no sisters. I had no idea what was "appropriate" for being a girl. By high school, my 5'8" tall, thick frame was constantly being called out as not attractive or feminine looking by all the boys. I had no idea how much all of this would negatively impact my life in the future as a wife, mother, and woman, but it certainly did.

I met my husband in 1999. We were both living it up, partying, and were in no way committed or in love. Within months of meeting, we found out we were having a child together, something that as I write cannot begin to capture the sheer terror we had around having an unplanned child at such a young age, let alone one together while not being in love. We did what we thought we "should" do and got married the following year after our daughter was born. We went on to welcome a second child in 2004 and a son in 2011.

Our marriage and family had been fairly stable for the first four years, but by 2005 things had become so incredibly tumultuous between us, we couldn't even stand each other or be around one another. The way we came together as a couple and the terrible conditions we had reached, led to the most devastating experience as a woman I have ever experienced to date.

In 2006, my husband came to me and told me he had had several affairs through the course of 2004-2006. I had been hearing this voice in my head saying *he's cheating* and had vaguely brought it up once, but never really pushed to know. He courageously had chosen to come out with it on his own. While this was single-handedly one of the most devastating times of my life, it was also the time the feminine side of who I was awakened and began showing up. The wounded feminine, as if to say *eff* you to all the men who had ever objectified me or shamed me for how I looked or acted most of my life.

This experience with infidelity shined a light on exactly how I had always felt about myself. I was determined to prove just how pretty, sexy, and desirable I was to a man. I wanted power over them subconsciously. I did not understand at the time that not aligning with my heart and soul before acting would cause my entire life to go completely out of whack for years afterward and if I had been patient and listened to my intuition, I would have been guided to a more peaceful and loving journey.

It started with extreme exercise. I began running 30+ miles a week just to escape. It felt so good to release the pain I was feeling through physical exertion. The running, at first, was medicine. It felt like I was being given this as a gift to help heal, and looking back it was exactly that. But something shifted when I started receiving a lot of attention for how my body looked. My ego began to show up in full form. I was being told I was skinny, or my hips were small or how fit I was looking. The attention felt incredible. It was like being seen for the very first time in a way I had never been seen before, but always wished I had. It was like I was being approved of as a *real* woman for the first time in my life. And so, the addiction began.

I eventually ended up getting into weight training and spending hours and hours a week in the gym to manipulate my body to stand out and less time running. So much of this time frame was deeply subconscious.

I was operating asleep by this point. It was like all the intuitive nudges that had always been there were now muted by the addiction from the pain I was trying to numb. Nonetheless, I did become addicted to the validation, but not just any validation. I became addicted to the validation by men and only men. It was like the more men I could get to look my way, the more sexy, powerful, and important I felt, so it's no surprise I ended up having several affairs of my own, something that shamed me deeply for years. This needs to be a chapter all on its own on the damage of cheating and affairs to a person, not just a marriage.

A couple of years later by January 2013, I had enrolled in a Life Coaching Certification program and by April that year, I had opened my own business helping women stuck in the diet culture, which at the time seemed fitting since I was all about health, even if I had a misconstrued idea of it at the time. I desperately wanted this business to save me from the darkness, the sadness, and the void I was living with inside. The void of no true self-respect or no true self-love. This was when my intuition started whispering to me. Between the constant need for validation and the affairs I had, I felt black inside. I had become so incredibly good at leaving the house all put together, looking the part for a man, but unable to be in silence or able to look at myself in the mirror. I knew there had to be more to life.

I spent the next five years struggling to make my business work and grow, with little to no success. I could never understand what was so off. I couldn't make things work or find the energy to stay consistent. By the end, I was exhausted. I had spent so much time and energy trying to make this work to save me I felt I had aged ten years and, to be honest, I had. My body didn't look the same as it used to and I felt things beginning to slip away. By 2018, five years after opening my doors I decided to close them feeling completely defeated. These five years were the most stubborn ever! I mean ever! I could hear my intuition whispering to me, it was there. It had started with a whisper here and there but by the end of 2018, it was getting louder and louder. *But I would not surrender.* I was so afraid of losing the false identity I had created that had given me attention and false validation in hopes the business would save me from myself and my behaviours. I had been living with hearing, "You're hot," "Wow, you opened your own business!" "Wow, look at your body!" "Wow, look at your fancy life in California." How could I let this false identity go? If I did, would I become nothing, or worse, would I die?

After closing my business painfully and resentfully, it wasn't long before I became involved in a few hobby-based businesses to keep me distracted and busy. None of which lasted and by 2019 I was in the most pain I had ever experienced to date. My intuition was literally, I mean literally screaming at me to *just take the mask and bandage off*! But still, I would not surrender.

In 2018-2019, our family had gone through a few very difficult situations with losing our beloved pastor to suicide, losing both our beloved pets tragically, and leaving our family home with a plan to move to another city and start a new life. All of which our family felt very emotional over. Between having a marriage brought together by a child and not being in love, infidelity on both sides and years of no self-love or self-respect for myself, our foundation made of quicksand had finally begun to sink and expose all the darkness in the wounded woman I was living as. The woman who had spent years operating asleep, unaware, and unconscious of her truth, and the truth. It was like watching it happen in slow motion and yet this time, I couldn't stop it.

First, I began drinking to numb the pain, something I *never* did before nor agreed with normally in my life. Then I turned to marijuana to see if this would work in drowning the pain out, again something I never did or agreed with before. Again, it didn't work. Then, I fell back into an old affair, and this was the final straw that led me over the edge to thoughts of suicide. If I could go back to an affair, with someone I didn't even love or truly want, if I could look to a man again for validation then what was I even worth anymore? Who was I if I wasn't sexy anymore? Who would I be if I didn't have a business anymore? Who was I if my husband and I weren't ever deeply in love and connected? My life fell apart and all of this happened right in front of my children. I had been walking around in front of them for most of their life asleep as a woman, asleep as a mother, and asleep as a wife. It had become so bad I wasn't even feeling anything like I should for my three incredible children I had been so blessed with by God, along with the supportive, loving husband (no matter his infidelities), and the life so many envied around me. I felt sick. Completely numb.

The summer of 2019 was the darkest time of my life, and it was also a time of reflection for my soul to find the light. While my life was crumbling, my oldest daughter fell into severe psychosis. I cannot describe, as a mother, the feeling of watching your child suffer the way my child did. The fear for all of us overcame all of our life circumstances.

I no longer needed to force, rush, fake, pretend, act, put on a show, please anyone or perform.

While as painful as this was, it was also the very best thing that could have ever happened to me as a mother, wife, and woman. It woke me up *finally*. I could see what I was doing right in front of her, and it brought me back to life. It brought me back to the light. *It saved me!*

By the end of 2019, I had started journaling systematically each day after hearing about a challenge Rachel Hollis had done with three things a day you journal, except I coined mine as "Four a Day Keeps The Negative Away." I had also heard from Lisa Nichols's book, No Matter What, that having a practice around gratitude helped to strengthen "the gratitude muscle." I also started meditating after reading the incredible book, Untethered Soul, and taking a course by Joe Dispenza called, Rewired, on why meditation is so powerful. And lastly, I started a small challenge online with women to do the same as I had started doing hoping this would help me have accountability. And it all began happening in a way that was coming from my heart and soul. A way I had been dreaming of. I began hearing my intuition more and more and this is where the calling for ayahuasca and plant medicine started to come in.

At the beginning of 2020, I decided to give my business one more try, a new fresh try, knowing I was coming from a different place. I don't think I fully understood this at the time but it was like I wanted to save women, but I hadn't even fully saved myself yet, or even learned how. Nonetheless, I had to do it, I had to go *through* it. I hired amazing coaches, went online, and started to get to work in a very masculine, very do, do, do kind of way.

I had decided no matter what I did with my business I would continue on the self-development path to reconnecting with my soul. I had signed up for a psilocybin healing ceremony and Tony Robbins's, Unleash The Power Within, event. Then, the pandemic hit, and both in-person events were cancelled. Tony Robbins decided to host his first virtual, Unleash The Power Within, and I was able to attend that, whereas the psilocybin ceremony healer had helped me begin a micro-dosing psilocybin regime while the event was on pause. Important side notes: I still to this day say the psilocybin micro-dosing ignited my brain to be able to reset old, unwanted patterns and truly woke me up.

I have always had this special love for mushrooms, very specifically psilocybin. As a young kid, I did "shrooms" (the street term for psilocybin) many times and felt universal shifts and always said if I could go back and safely, responsibly go there again as an adult, I would. In other words, I always knew they had a special connection for me.

I spent almost all of 2020 building and growing my business and working on myself from a deep place within. I had started to succeed in the way I thought I wanted to financially. Yet, I still didn't feel fulfilled. I didn't understand how I had gotten what I had asked for financially without feeling satisfied by it all. I knew very quickly if I resisted this time and did not listen to my intuition I could lose my life, fall to the ground, or at the very least repeat the cycle all over again.

In October 2020, a chain of "coincidental" networking conversations happened to lead me to connect with a healer who works with plant medicine. Specifically, ayahuasca and psilocybin. I had seen a noticeable difference in the ability to connect to my intuition throughout the year with the help of micro-dosing psilocybin, self-development tools and the spiritual work through meditation and journaling, etc. but I did feel something was missing and there was more I needed. So, in December 2020, I committed to my first ayahuasca ceremony, scheduled for January 2021.

I had no idea that 2021 would be the year of waking to my full intuition. I could write an entire book on the first ayahuasca journey I did in January 2021. I received clarity and messages that I would be working as a healer, my husband was indeed the love of my life, and some incredibly deep ancestral healing received extended to my parents. It was a life-changing experience.

Upon arriving home after the first ceremony my husband felt in complete awe of the transformation he saw happen right in front of him and felt called to a journey of his own. So in March 2021, he and I, as well as some friends came together and went into what was now ceremony number two for me. I cannot speak about my husband's journey, but once again in this ceremony I received continued confirmation that I had received from ceremony number one, as well as deep, deep healing between my husband and me around the years of infidelity, the years living with a lack of love for each other, the conditioning we both came into the relationship with as a man and a woman, and most of all the ancestral healing through generations of conditioning and programming we both had been living with. It was incredibly healing for both my husband and I individually, and as a couple.

Following ceremony number two, I went back to resume business as usual but this time there was this sensation in my body I had not felt before. It was almost like my body had a braking system. I would go to work with clients with marketing or promoting and there was this organic brake happening where I could not make my body do what did not feel right. I listened and started to set fire to anything I had already built or that did not feel aligned, and I did it unapologetically. Many around me didn't understand. They questioned and judged me, but I knew I had to do it regardless and I was going to fully surrender. It was finally time.

I call the end of 2021 The Beautiful Colourful Fire.

The business I had built was full of colour, full of depth, full of options and extremely saturated in boldness. It was a stunning "looking" online business. By the summer of 2021, I had started to build my most beautiful masterpiece in an online coaching program to help women free themselves from diet culture. I had always felt this calling to help women live free from a diet and in fact, I despised dieting all my life after witnessing my mother struggle her whole life with diets. But something happened in the first two ceremonies where I felt this chain *finally* break as if to say, "Saving women from dieting is not your burden to carry anymore, let it go." When I started to build this program, it almost felt like the old me putting a bow on top of a box I would then lovingly place on a shelf like you would a collectible, and theoretically, that is precisely what I did. I completed the program in September 2021, stopped all activity in the business and went silent. *Silent* in a way I could hear a pin drop in all areas of my life. I no longer needed to force, rush, fake, pretend, act, put on a show, please anyone or perform. I was ready to just be and watch the beautiful fire be set to my beloved business and all it had done to help carry me through the years I refused to listen. I had held on so tight to my ego and would never surrender to my deeper calling from God. It was like watching a field be set on fire and the flames were so vibrant with colour you couldn't even speak a word (the field of flames being your past being burned away).

The Reflection of My Reflection

As I write this, it is December 2021. I completed my third and final ceremony of the year. This ceremony was different this time. This ceremony wasn't about healing, it was about being initiated into the calling I've been running from. A calling that has scared me all my life. A calling that caused judgment to be passed on me so hard I had dimmed my light and begged it to stop and go away. A calling that is beyond any words or language available to me here on earth. And a calling that when I listen to and follow leads me to completeness so unexplainable, I can only say, thank you, God.

I have a gift with intuition and when I show up fully, allowing my intuition or spirit to move through me, she brings me to the most beautiful space I have ever felt in my life. A whole woman, a pure woman, and a healed feminine and masculine woman. This intuition shows the illumination in others and a never-ending understanding of their darkness. I am unclear today as I write this where I will be led with this gift, but all I know is that it cannot be rushed and I am to remain focused, calm, and in complete gratitude.

As I said at the very beginning of this chapter, if the younger version of me had a glimpse at the current circumstances without knowing the whole story, she would have freaked the hell out! Whereas, I sit here today full of gratitude for this new chance and opportunity in life. I no longer feel stuck in the rat race, in a program as a woman, living in conditions being passed down on me or expected of me. I am no longer living to please a man. I am simply being present, day by day, allowing this Godly intuition to guide me in a whole way to the place it has shown me. I could have never imagined that removing the band-aid and slowing things down could have brought me to such a place of happiness and love. I am eternally grateful for this and for the new chapter given to me, coming from a whole place, filled with spirit. For this is what I have always longed for.

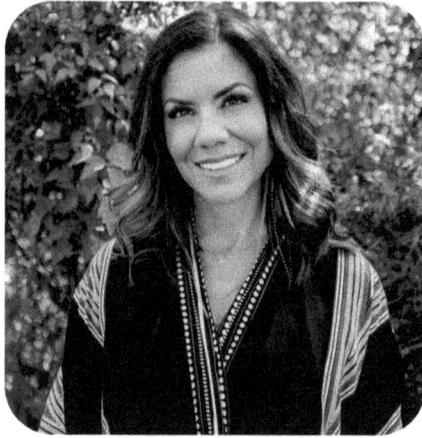

Jeanette Lucero

Jeanette Lucero is a wife and mother of three living in the sunny Southern California area, originally from Albuquerque, NM. She's spent over twenty years dedicated to health and wellness and almost ten of those years serving women as a Mindset Health Coach. She helps women release the diet mindset through her business 85/15 Lifestyle. She is a certified Life Coach, Personal Trainer and Nutrition Consultant.

Jeanette's family is the centre of her heart and everyday focus. She loves being a mother to her three children Samantha 21, Montessa 17, and Ambrose 10. Her twenty-year plus marriage to her husband John continues to be a priority and heart-centred focus towards the growth and happiness of the marriage.

Her hobbies and interests include anything physical, yoga, running, weight training, hiking, and reading. Spending time with her plant collection, travelling and educating herself on all the different healing modalities used in the healing world.

After attending three ayahuasca ceremonies in 2020 in search of a deeper understanding and meaning to life, Jeanette's professional path as a health coach took a drastic turn into the healing world. She currently is immersed in her studies around healing modalities with a specific focus on plant medicines such as psilocybin. This new path has her very excited for the future in serving others through natural healing methods and she looks forward to utilizing the knowledge in the future.

I would love to take this special opportunity to give thanks and gratitude to my always supportive husband John and our three children Samantha, Montessa and Ambrose. They have been the constant in my life and never-ending love. They are my all. I love each of you guys most!

CHAPTER SEVEN

The Broken Boy

Kary Odiatu

I will let fall a shower of roses. I will spend my heaven doing good on earth.

-St. Therese (The Little Flower)

These are the words on my son's gravestone. A message I hope to carry forward in my life. Inspiring people to take action with their health and to be so grateful for what they have been given. That is the gift my firstborn gave me. I haven't spoken publicly about the days surrounding his death at the age of eight in 2013. And in the initial writing attempts for *Every Body Holds a Story*, I purposely avoided this topic, flirting with inspirational messages instead. The stress of the covid pandemic had limited my creative intuition and thinking about the past seemed like a bad idea when I was having a hard time focusing on being present.

You know those days when you are frazzled and can't concentrate or even stroke one item off your to-do list? Well, I had been having one of those months. Higher than normal anxiety levels were creeping up stealthily like a cat on the prowl. My daily exercise routine and nature walks were not cutting it anymore. Have you ever experienced physical signs that your body is in constant fight or flight? The pressure within my throat and heart centre was unbearable at times. It was time for a reset—time for spiritual help.

I headed to my Reiki healer for an energy treatment; hoping to gain some peace of mind and some clarity for writing. I am not usually one who is lacking in stories to tell yet choosing the right story for this chapter of my life wasn't happening. As I pulled up in front of her house I received a text from a friend who is a scientific researcher in a company that works in genome sequencing. We hadn't talked about my son in years, so I was surprised to read her message. She asked if Jordan, who was born with severe Lissencephaly (smooth brain) ever had whole-genome sequencing or genetic testing. Her company would be running tests on unsolved genetic cases at the Toronto Hospital for Sick Kids. I immediately felt triggered reading the message. I didn't need this extra stress as I was heading in for my Reiki treatment, hoping to figure out what I needed to write about. I quickly replied I did not want to dredge up the past as they never did discover any genetic reason for his condition and I had conveniently "compacted" that time of my life into a small folder in my brain somewhere that I only occasionally peek at.

I was a few minutes early for my appointment, so I went to that folder in my mind and took a glimpse inside. The amount of guilt a parent has when a child is born with a birth defect or disorder is indescribable. *It can eat you alive.* I spent so many hours running through a "guilt trip list" I had created in my head. Regularly reviewing it and adding more items as I pondered what I had done to cause this condition my child was born with. Maybe it was the glass of wine I drank, maybe it was the stress of the across-country move we made when he was conceived, maybe it was all the supplements and protein shakes I had taken during ten years of professional athleticism in the sport of women's fitness. I could feel the judgment from friends and family who didn't understand my dedication to my sport, let alone my decision to wait until my mid-thirties to start a family. These judgments were articulated by a social worker soon after my son's birth. She asked me if the "extreme" exercise I continued to do while pregnant may have contributed to the lack of the baby's brain development. I will never forget this moment as long as I live. I screamed at her to, "*GET OUT!*" of my hospital room. I chased her out the door. Nurses came running to calm me down as I screamed what that monster had said to me. She later asked to come and apologize—I refused to see her and allow her that absolution. To this day I carry a little guilt that I could not accept her apology. And, in my own, *I'll show them*, way, I went on to have four more healthy children (two in my forty's) and maintained a similar workout routine with each pregnancy to prove her accusations were unfounded. In hindsight, I'm sure she was voicing what many in my life were thinking.

It was a long time before I was able to give myself grace and toss that invisible list of blame. Jordan only lived for eight years, although living through it felt like an eternity some days. Especially the days when I had no other help and another crying newborn to attend to. Those days when I would be out for a quick errand and wouldn't want to return home. I'm sure every mom has these feelings at some point in the overwhelm of being the lighthouse for everyone else. I gave up a speaking career requiring a lot of travel, which I loved, because of panic attacks and my need to stay close to my healthy children.

I took a deep breath and headed in for my Reiki treatment. I could feel the tightness in my chest and the congestion in my body as she started the treatment. Not the kind you get from a cold but the kind that comes with stress. An all too familiar feeling. I knew my adrenals were fatigued and my energy was not flowing freely. As I entered deep into a meditative state, I could slowly feel my body releasing tension. My mind drifted as I focused on my deep breathing. Then I saw a bonfire with red-golden flames dancing in the shadows. Across the bonfire was one of my spiritual gurus who is no longer alive in the physical sense but repeatedly comes to me in visions and dreams, Dr. Wayne Dyer. He is bare-footed and wearing a black cap and sweater. I slowly let my gaze flow to the left and there is my mom in a lawn chair wrapped up in a cozy blanket. She passed away before the pandemic in January 2020. I turn my head to my right and my departed son Jordan is sitting in his wheelchair with a big smile on his face enjoying the sparks of light thrown off the fire.

I begin to think to myself, *I am surrounded by dead people,* yet they are as real to me as they were when they were physically alive. Another shadow steps into the scene and it is the Catholic priest who buried my son. I am a little shocked to see him as he is still alive as far as I know and I'm a little amused as well since my mom is one of the most anti-establishment people I know. She was not fond of churches and formal religion—to put it nicely. I looked at Wayne and asked him, "What do you have for me today, Wayne?" He smiled and started reciting the Lord's prayer. I couldn't hear all of the words when I remembered I was in a meditation, and I probably wouldn't be able to complete the prayer without googling it since it had been close to forty years since the daily repetition in elementary school. That's when the Catholic priest joined in and I found myself reciting the lines along with them.

> Our Father who art in heaven
> Hallowed be thy Name,
> Thy kingdom come,
> Thy will be done,
> On earth, as it is in heaven.
> Give us this day our daily bread.
> And forgive us our trespasses,
> As we forgive those who trespass against us.
> And lead us not into temptation,
> But deliver us from evil.
> For thine is the kingdom,
> And the power, and the glory,
> Forever and ever. Amen.

As the words of the Lord's prayer ran through my head, I felt a huge wave of release wash over my body and tears began to stream from my eyes. The congestion left my chest and nasal passages, and I knew my friend's text that morning and my vision were gentle nudges from the Universe that it was time to stop running from the past. Time to share my experience of my son's passing away. Time to do some good on earth during a time when many people are feeling broken.

I will never forget the beginning of the end for my son. It was

Valentine's Day 2013, and I was sitting in foils in my hairdresser's chair getting my hair done for a night out. My phone rang and it was the supervisor of the people who helped care for my son. She never called unless there was an emergency, and she had never asked me to come right away before. It could always wait. This time was different. Her voice was different. She told me it would be a good idea to come as soon as possible. Jordan had taken a turn for the worse with the cold he had and was having a lot of difficulty clearing his lungs. I immediately called his physiotherapist who had become like family and started to cry. I had a feeling we would not be able to turn it around this time. The doctors had told us we would be lucky if he lived to age two. He was now eight years young and permanently connected to oxygen to help him breathe. We knew a respiratory illness would be the last straw for his weak system that had been medicated and g-tube fed for eight years. His condition deteriorated quickly and in a panic, we rushed him to Sick Kids even though hospitalization and extreme measures were not part of his end-of-life plan to pass peacefully at home surrounded by loved ones. No matter how much you think you are prepared for the death of a loved one—you have no clue how you will feel or react when that time draws near.

I sat in Sick Kids hospital late that night in my son's dark room wanting desperately to get him back home. I was stuck to my chair engulfed in tears and guilt and uncertainty, questioning if I was doing the right thing by caring for him at home. That's when the most amazing miracle happened that I will never forget. Someone must have contacted our palliative care doctor because he magically appeared in my son's hospital room late at night, on a weekend. He looked me in the eye and asked me to remember what our plan was for Jordan and his end of life. I said, "He should be at home, but I am terrified and what if the hospital could do something for him that we couldn't." He reassured me Jordan's caregivers were very well prepared and there was nothing the hospital could do for him that we couldn't do. He gave me permission to stick to my plan. An angel in disguise sent, in one of my darkest hours. He told me to get my boy home and he would assign a doctor to us for in-home palliative support. I breathed a sigh of relief knowing in my heart and gut that it was the right thing to do. I did not want my boy to pass away in a hospital bed. I called one of his caregivers and two showed up with the wheelchair van to help transport him home. We hummed the Mission Impossible theme music as we scooted his wheelchair out of Sick Kids hospital, zig-zagging the halls to "sneak him out."

Jordan's father was raised in a strong Catholic family, so I agreed to a Catholic end of life. It didn't matter to me as I felt that once Jordan was "gone" he would be a child of the Universe/God force no matter what happened. We called in a Catholic priest to perform Last Rights over him. I have never been a religious/church person and prefer to call myself "spiritual" rather than use a label to categorize into any one religion. Yet this Catholic priest had a special energy about him and I connected with him immediately. He asked me about Jordan and Jordan's caregivers and his brief life. He listened intently as I painted the picture of all the amazing people that had come into our lives because of Jordan.

The next day I arranged for a dear friend to help me pick up some groceries for my nanny and the kids; I couldn't be alone. I felt I would lose it if left alone. My friend needed something in the next aisle and disappeared for a brief moment. I froze in the aisle unable to move, tears streaming down my face as the words, *broken boy*, ran through my mind. My child is broken and I couldn't fix him. No matter how hard I tried and now he is going to die. I'm not sure how long I stood there frozen in the aisle until my friend came back to gently escort me out and back to my broken boy. I do remember wailing in her embrace before going back into the house.

Jordan Daniel Odiatu passed away in my arms at the age of 8, on February 16th, 2013.

The days following were a blur of doing the unthinkable. . . planning a funeral for a child. A being you had birthed into the world. As a parent, you never expect to outlive your child. I sat in the pews at my son's funeral a few short days later, still filled with the angst of loss after eight years of doing my best to keep my little man alive. Wondering how a priest I had only recently met could possibly deliver a message about a broken boy he hardly knew. A boy who had been unable to run, walk, play, eat by mouth, sit or stand. He started speaking about our family, Jordan, and his caregivers with words that anyone could have spoken. Then my head snapped up in attention as he said the following words:

*"Jordan was **broken** in a sense, unable to enter into many of the usual things of childhood and youth. Even breathing was a*

struggle for Jordie. Yet he moved hearts. His smile was infectious. He was blessed with a unique ability to awaken our hearts, to draw us together around him so that his blessing became our blessing and our humanity blossomed in his presence. Perhaps we could learn through him something utterly simple about God's shaping our life stories. Like the bread at Eucharist, we too are taken by God, each life chosen for a particular and unique purpose. Like the bread and Jordie, each of us is blessed in different ways, with talents, friends, grace, and hunger to live with love. Like bread, each of us is broken somewhere in life—where we run into failure or darkness or some shadow."

I had a moment alone with the Catholic Priest after the service. I looked deep into his eyes and told him about my experience with *the broken boy* dialogue in the grocery store. He smiled knowingly when I asked him how he decided to speak about the topic of the broken boy for my son's funeral. He told me he had been in angst for a while over what to say at a child's funeral. The most difficult funeral. He had prayed for a long time and the broken boy message had come to him clearly in prayer. The goosebumps sprung to attention on my arms, and I jokingly said I was thinking of becoming Catholic. The priest chuckled and we hugged, and I knew my son, the priest, and I had somehow connected on a level beyond the physical, beyond the labels of religion, to deliver a message to others that could offer hope and consolation in times of great darkness. As Joel Osteen says,

"The brokenness is not the end. It is a sign that God is about to multiply. The more broken you are, the more God is going to increase. Don't focus on what you have lost—focus on what you still have. There is strength in all the broken pieces."

As I saw the people who had gathered to remember my son and support my family, I knew this was true. We were all broken fragments of the Universe brought together because of my son. We all will feel broken at some point. Broken promises, broken dreams, broken hearts, broken marriages. I had wanted a baby so bad and all the things that come with being a mom. Mom and baby classes, long stroller walks and playdates with other moms. I lost all of that when my medically fragile and complex care baby was born. Yet, somehow, I gained so much more.

"When you change the way you look at things, the things you look at change."

-Dr. Wayne Dyer

People have often asked me how I was able to get on with my life. How I was able to still laugh and live my best life and trust enough to have four more babies after losing my first. One of my favourite authors, Dr. Wayne Dyer, once spoke of what comes out when you squeeze an orange? Simply—orange juice. No matter what happens in your life or how you get squeezed, what is inside will come out. When you hit the hard breaks in life you will be squeezed and this is your chance to

Tapping into trapped emotions is important because emotion is energy in the body and this energy can become congested if not released.

examine what is coming out. To deal with that. To release what is not you and make a conscious choice on how you respond. I decided I was not going to get bitter. I was not going to give up on my hopes and dreams. I would focus on the **gifts** from Jordan's life, not the trials. Based on the work of Joe Dispenza, "If you can't find the lessons and gifts—your body will continue living in the same experience." Every time an emotion arises you are running off the memories of the past. Things are constantly changing and the central force to emotional stability and happiness is not having control over change, rather it is choosing to be in the *now*. Or more concretely, finding the gifts at any moment, *right here, right now*. Ask yourself: am I trying to change this or is this a gift?

This is how you train your body to have a different response in emotional situations that dredge up memories or physiology.

Music plays a powerful role in my healing and in my ability to connect deeply to my feelings which I can easily avoid as I am a naturally joyful person that gravitates towards fun. Tapping into trapped emotions is important because emotion is energy in the body and this energy can become congested if not released. Flipping the scripts allows us to run through our minds on repeat and look for examples of how others have successfully done this is something else I focus on in my daily life. It is a gift to know that everything is happening *for* you, not to you. I'll never forget the time Prince performed the halftime show at the Super Bowl. It had been raining cats and dogs and the organizers asked Prince if he was ok. He replied, "Can you make it rain harder?" It was magic—a stadium full of people united as they crooned the lyrics of Purple Rain in the pouring rain. In an interview, Prince was asked the meaning of the song Purple Rain and he replied, "When there's blood in the sky, red + blue = purple. . . purple rain pertains to the end of the world and being with the one you love and letting your faith/god guide you through the purple rain." A perfect example of turning life's storms into opportunities to rise up and grow. I played this song while I stared at the outline of a leafless, dead tree in the drizzle on the day before my son died. Any time I need an emotional decongestion it's one of my go-to tools.

Having a child opens your heart like nothing else I have ever experienced. Losing a child rips your heart right out of your chest. I have read that after carrying your baby for nine months, fragments of their DNA will stay in your body forever. I always feel that Jordan is with me—even if he is not physically with me. My son is my screensaver on my phone. Seeing him every day reminds me to fall in love with being alive. To be grateful for my body that can walk, run, dance, jump, my arms that can hug and write, my mouth that can talk and eat. Each day I give thanks and never take any of this for granted.

> *"Lighten your heart by engaging in enjoyable activities: sing, dance, watch the sunset, take a nap or hug someone with exuberance."*
>
> *-Doreen Virtue*

Before Jordan, I used to think a healthy lifestyle was the answer to every problem. I had a hard time connecting to people on more than a surface level—I had a lot of success—but not a lot of depth. Because of Jordan I became more compassionate and had more empathy for others and saw this in every caregiver and friend and family member that spent time with my son. Have you ever noticed this in your life? A group that includes someone who requires more care is often more caring and inclusive. I have seen this throughout the years as a teacher and as a coach. Classes with special needs children in them were always the best classes with the most conscientious children. I will never forget a special child named Shea in a grade four class when I was a gym teacher. We were playing a game of soccer baseball and Shea kicked the ball and started to run in the wrong direction. All the kids in the class cheered him on and proceeded to purposely miss every throw attempt to get him out. Shea rounded the bases and the whole class celebrated with him as he arrived home. I have seen this with my children as well. My eldest daughter went to school with a girl in a wheelchair from kindergarten through to grade eight. That group of kids was a very kind group that never needed adult intervention for bullying or mean girl behaviour.

"The moment can define you, or you can define the moment."

-Eric Worre

I went through a dark night of the soul, and I survived and chose to thrive. I had to become an advocate for my son who did not have a voice. I had to come to terms with death and dying and was able to talk about that to Jordan's sisters who were six and four at the time of his passing. We spoke of the lifecycle of a leaf and family pets. Concrete examples in our lives that everything has a life cycle and in the falling of the leaf lies the opportunity for new growth as the leaf breaks down to become part of the soil which will eventually sprout a new tree or feed another human or animal. Not lost or gone—just a shift in how it is expressed or experienced. Like this story keeps the spirit of my son *alive* in a sense. When you confront death early in life you realize you can spend your life running from death or running towards life and the extreme gratitude for life is directly related to living in the *right here—right now* finding magic moments in every moment.

I now have my dream of being a mom to three healthy little girls and little brother Theo who was born two years after Jordan passed. These children gained a very patient mom. No matter what happens, or what they do, I am always thankful they are alive. I know I treat them all with a deeper sense of respect and awareness, knowing how fleeting life is. I gained a support network of amazing people, some of whom are still dear friends to this day. The magic moments that happened along the way, the angels that come into our lives in physical form, the nurse who let me sleep in the cot in the nurse's sleeping room because I refused to leave the hospital while my son was in the NICU, the nurse who whispered in my ear Jordan needed to be in Sick Kids Hospital downtown where they had specialists to treat him properly and rooms I could stay in with him, the caregivers that treated him like one of their own family members, and the ones that did not leave at the end of my son's life—even when their shifts ended. The list of magic moments is long.

I had to come to terms that he was perfect as he was and to see the beauty in the brokenness. I have always loved collecting sea glass at the beach and often think of Jordan when I find a special piece, especially the blue pieces because they are rare, like he was. Every time a blue jay lands in my backyard I remember his soul is flying like those birds, free of the physical limitations he was born with.

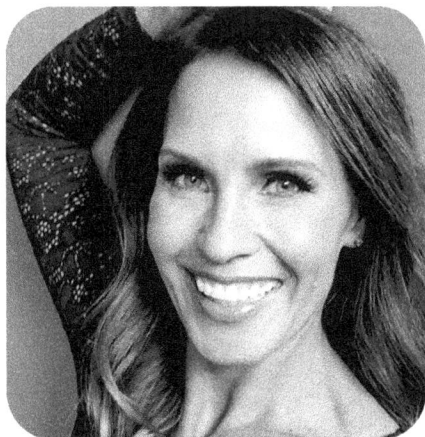

Kary Odiatu

Kary Odiatu, BEd. , BPE, Certified Trainer & Nutritional Consultant. Co-author of Fit For the LOVE of It! And The Miracle of Health (2009 Harper Collins). Kary resides in Unionville, ON and is a Mom of four school-age kids. She operates a successful home-based business in the Health and Wellness space. Kary represented Canada internationally as a women's fitness competitor for ten years, competing at the prestigious Fitness Olympia and Arnold Sports Festival. She has co-authored two books and has lectured on health and wellness throughout Canada and the United States. Kary is passionate about inspiring others to take action with their health and is always looking at the big picture when it comes to optimal strategies for function, healthy aging, independence and well-being. She is also a certified Heal Your Life Teacher, through Hay House and the work of Louise Hay. Her mantra is: Make Life Magical and she believes there are *no excuses* when it comes to staying **fit and having fun**!

IG @karyodiatu

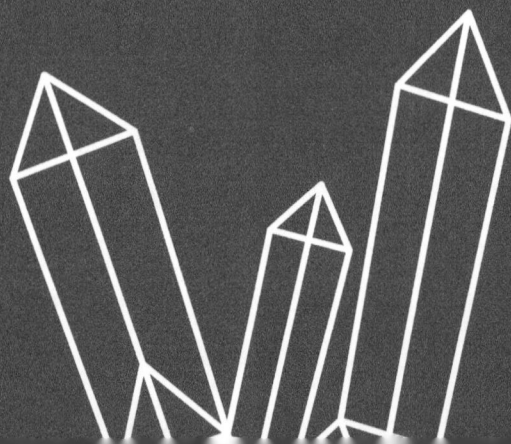

CHAPTER EIGHT

Your Sign For Self Advocation

Aujha Hastings

"I'm sorry babe, it just feels like nails; nails are scratching my insides every time we have sex," I said this at the beginning of May 2016, for the fifth time that year, to my now ex-boyfriend. We only had sex about once a month due to the immense pain and this is how I felt every single time. It may have been more than that, especially if I felt guilty, but that's a ballpark guess because in the grand scheme of things, once a month was not often in my opinion. *(A friendly reminder—and a reminder to myself—we should never feel guilty for not having sex when we don't want to).*

This is where it all began though, with the pain. The nails scratching me internally. It was every time. Every damn time. But do you think I made a doctor's appointment? No way, I was "too busy" for that. That is until the pain became something I could no longer ignore, even when walking around. What started with pain strictly during sex, turned into a constant twinge in my pelvic region.

The additional pain started near the end of May 2016 and progressively got worse. My first visit to my family doctor was on June 14th. He asked me a bunch of questions and did an impromptu pap test to see if it came back with anything. He said he would send off a referral to a gynecologist to look into this further for me. At the very least, that day I felt relieved to feel like I was going to figure out why I was in such constant pain. As the days went on without answers and the pain gradually increased, there was comfort in knowing I was headed in the right direction. This was the worst pain I had ever experienced (at that point in my life) and I wouldn't wish it upon anyone.

As a hairstylist, I began my career working for a salon in downtown London, Ontario long before going to hair school. I officially joined as a full-time stylist (and desk coordinator) in November 2015 upon graduation from the Aveda Academy in Toronto. In May 2016, I had just turned twenty-four years old, I was still in my first year of client-building, working my ass off, and plagued with constant pain. I was concerned about what this would mean in terms of appointments with doctors, considering that asking for time off during the first year as a stylist when you're at the bottom of the proverbial food chain, was hard to achieve. I know doctor appointments shouldn't be a worry, but I also wondered about time for personal events.

I was eight months into what I like to refer to as my "big girl" job and I was grateful I was allowed to leave early on June 23rd, 2016, for my stepdad's birthday dinner. Birthdays are a big deal in my family and whenever possible, I try to be there for everyone's big day. I have a great relationship with my stepdad, so, on his birthday I felt tremendous guilt for feeling relieved about leaving work early, only to miss his dinner and drive myself to the Urgent Care Center at one of London's hospitals. This was the closest hospital to the salon, and I didn't want to sit for hours on end in the ER at another hospital located in the south end of the city. My pelvic pain was *so* terrible that I couldn't go to dinner, and I couldn't sit at home and hope for the pain to pass.

Unfortunately, they couldn't do much during that hospital visit other than send me home without answers, just the standard, "Take Tylenol and Advil on rotation to help manage the pain and come back if it gets worse." Well, at that point Tylenol and Advil were not cutting it for me at all, and work was becoming a daunting task to stand and talk with clients pretending everything was normal all day long.

After a week had passed, my boss took me back to the same hospital and waited with me until my mom could get there. I had to leave in the middle of a haircutting class because I couldn't bear to sit there, and the word *pain* really did not describe the havoc my body was enduring. Amongst my physical agony, while waiting with my boss for the triage nurse to call me, I did get a good laugh with her about my name. It's not one you'd hear anywhere you go and the poor nurse reading "Aujha" out loud for someone she didn't know would be a challenging task for anyone. I've been on the receiving end of these name attempts my entire life and if anyone said anything that started or ended with an "a" or "aw" sound, I recognized it as me.

"Oi-Ya?" I immediately jumped to my feet. "How do you know that's you?" My boss asked, amused. "I just do," I replied, with a slight shrug of the shoulders and a smile on my face, grateful for the moment of positivity.

When I was triaged and sent back to sit with my boss, she asked, "So do you just stand up to any weird sound when you're waiting for something like this? In any given scenario?" I replied, "Yeah, pretty much. After a while, you get used to it and realize they're calling you. That's why at Starbucks I always say my name is Amanda." We laughed, in a hospital waiting room with the perfect distraction of discussing all the various pronunciations I've ever heard throughout my life. Laughter was exactly what I needed for my mental state at that moment.

> I honestly didn't know what to do for myself other than try to persevere through life and see if my pain would magically go away.

After being admitted and checked over, I left the hospital with no answers once again, feeling like I might have to live like this forever and feeling like I was just a gnat the doctors and nurses needed to swat away. I honestly didn't know what to do for myself other than try to persevere through life and see if my pain would magically go away. Feeling dismissed by a range of healthcare professionals, as well as family for being dramatic or having a low pain tolerance, I was overcome by a sense of loneliness and deflation.

At this point, I had received multiple transvaginal ultrasounds, abdominal ultrasounds, bloodwork, one pap test from my family doctor's office, answered a thousand questions, and ingested two Costco-sized bottles of painkillers that ultimately did nothing. The hospital also didn't think it was necessary to do another pap test only two weeks after I had one, which made sense to me at the time, but I was still frustrated and searching for a doctor or nurse who cared enough to dive deeper into my concerns about what was going on within my body. This pain was not normal, and I instinctively knew I needed a doctor's help—I needed to keep pushing. Simultaneously, I wondered what use it would do since I didn't have any answers or an appointment with the gyne-cologist referral yet.

Another week went by after this particular urgent care visit and after surviving six days of work, while attempting to maintain a social life, it was my sister's eighteenth birthday on July 7th. I toughed it out only to return to the ER. This time at the other hospital in the south end of the city, the very next day. A few people had suggested trying this hospital instead as there was a better and more informed gynecological team. This decision ultimately steered me in the right direction, and I wish I had gone sooner. The only reason I didn't was because of their insane wait times but the wait seemed worth it now after failing to manage the pain on my own.

As I waited to be admitted, I sat with my then ex-boyfriend for over six hours. I was simultaneously grateful for his support while we waited, plagued with stress over the toxicity of our relationship and wanting it to end. It felt like I had an immense weight sitting on my shoulders with all the unknowns in my life and my pelvic pain kept nagging me and taking over. I was about to crack under the pressure of it all and honestly, couldn't focus on anything else.

My ex had to leave for work just as I was put in a bed in the ER. I started from the beginning of my symptoms with the resident doctor on shift. They did more ultrasounds and ran more bloodwork. The resident was about to send me home when I begged for him to send a second referral to a gynecologist as well. They were very reluctant to do so because I was already waiting on an appointment from the referral my family doctor sent out but I begged and I begged and I begged. I absolutely could not go home feeling completely defeated again and feeling like I should have pushed harder for better care. The simple act of going home and thinking you *should* have done more or said more to get what you need from a healthcare worker is *far* worse than feeling like a crazy person for *actually* asking for it. Finally, he agreed and said their referral might come in sooner, which it did. My appointment was set for July 14th, 2016, less than a week later. Hallelujah!

I have so much gratitude for this gynecologist, Dr. One, and all of his compassion and hard work. When I went in for my appointment, he let me explain every single detail, asked me several questions, and offered to do another pap test because he wanted to be thorough and start fresh from the beginning while in his care. My pap test was done one month after my family doctor did one. *Thirty days.* He called me two days later and asked me to come in to discuss the results. As I sat in his office, he explained to me he would continue to investigate my pain but needed to refer me to a second gynecologist in London, Dr. Two, because I had second grade, high-risk, abnormal cervical cells from my pap test. In thirty days, I went from a clean test to second grade, high-risk cells. Queue the stress.

In addition to the discovery of these cells, Dr. One said he speculated endometriosis, but in my case, I couldn't be 100% diagnosed without laparoscopic surgery since nothing was discovered in any scans or pelvic exams. Endometriosis is a painful disorder where tissue similar to the tissue that lines your uterus, the endometrium, grows outside your uterus. It thickens, then breaks down and causes bleeding (just like it would in the uterus). He decided my first option for pain management was to start taking Visanne, a progestin that acts like progesterone (a specific, mainly female, hormone) in the body. Progestins reduce the effects of estrogen on tissues, such as the lining of the uterus. He said it was mainly intended to help subside my pain, but it can also essentially be a form of birth control without actually being birth control, as it may stop my cycle altogether and preserve my fertility—a big bonus in my opinion. I began taking the Visanne and was also recommended to a pelvic floor physiotherapist.

With newfound hope, this would soon be over, and I'd go back to living and working a normal life (minus the concern about the abnormal cells), I was able to enjoy dinner for my brother's birthday on July 18th. My family was happy that I was on a path to answers and so was I. My constant aches throughout dinner were soon going to be a thing of the past and things were looking up. The pain became somewhat manageable, and I was beginning to make it through full workdays and a social life. My newest worry though was the speculated endometriosis and what that might mean for my fertility, as it can potentially lead to problems. This led to a spiral of thoughts about my relationship and further increased my stress about wanting to leave.

By the end of July 2016, I finally ended my relationship, and by August 1st, I felt like a new woman! I began going out with friends and co-workers more frequently and experiencing a sense of freedom I had not felt in so long. The pain still lingered in the background but was no longer debilitating. My family doctor's referral had finally come through for the end of August and I happily declined as I was grateful for my care with Dr. One, as well as the Visanne that was helping me live more freely. I did prolong my pelvic floor physio appointment, due to lack of insurance coverage and because for the moment, I was feeling okay. I was even able to enjoy my dad's birthday at the beginning of October without any fear of missing it.

I don't know what changed but something ended up re-triggering my intense endometriosis pain and by November, I was calling Dr. One again. (Now that I've had a baby with a natural birth with no pain meds, after experiencing all this in 2016 I can confidently say my daily and constant pelvic pain was equivalent to the early stages of labour). At the beginning of November, I was in the office at work, laying on the floor between clients, calling in sick here and there to try and space it out, and finally calling for a pelvic floor physio appointment. My short little burst of fun, happiness and normalcy felt like it was coming to its end and the stress levels were on the rise again. Not to mention having to see Dr. Two for the abnormal pap test, which confirmed the same second-grade, high-risk cervical cells. They needed to repeat this pap in six months, which began the waiting game—my favourite.

By the end of November 2016, the Visanne was no longer keeping the pain at bay and I was calling my boss and requesting the rest of the week off to try and recoup myself. I also called Dr. One to request a surgery referral and explained I was now off work, and the pain was impeding my daily life. *(This was 100% true, but I later learned you have to actually say that for them to consider surgery, according to the surgeon).* Having to make that call to my boss to reschedule and push client appointments left me with a great level of devastation, completely indescribable. I knew I was letting my boss down by needing time off and the unknown of it was lingering in the back of my mind as I stressed about missing the busy Christmas season at the salon (which was prime client-building time). This ultimately created panic about my finances because I couldn't make money unless I was working. I didn't know if I would be able to work full days again and I had rent to pay, animals to feed, groceries to buy, a student loan to make payments on, car insurance, gas, utilities, etc. I also had a trip to Cuba planned for the middle of January, having booked it back in October when I was feeling good and making money to pay for it all! I officially became a couch potato, a very sad couch potato.

When Dr. One's office called me back to approve the referral request, they asked if there was anywhere, in particular, I wanted to go. I said, "I will fly to another province if it means they can do the surgery tomorrow."

By Monday, November 28th, a doctor in Stratford, Ontario, "Dr. Three," had his receptionist call and give me a date for Friday, December 16th, 2016. I said thank you a million times and breathed the biggest sigh of relief. About thirty seconds later, relief turned into panic as I realized I would be off work until just before Christmas. The anxiety around missing my career-building opportunity of the holiday season began to set in. I called Dr. Three's office and asked to be put on a cancellation list for anything sooner, I could be there at any given notice. They were very kind and added my name to the list. I knew it was a long shot to get in sooner, but you never know unless you ask. It was pretty miraculous that December 16th was available because I remember being told it can usually take a couple of months to get in.

All I wanted was to be and feel normal again. The stress of worrying about my finances and missing out on growing my clientele was no longer serving me so I did my absolute best to focus on what I wanted. Believe it or not, my thoughts worked and the very next day, Tuesday, November 29th, Dr. Three's office called and said they had a cancellation for *that* Friday, December 2nd. I was so excited, I immediately called my boss and told her the great news. I would simply need the weekend off for surgery and recovery and be back brand new by Monday, December 5th. She was kind and told me to take Monday and Tuesday off too, but I had already taken so many days off at that point I wanted to be back in the salon as soon as possible. Plus, I knew I would have to take another day off for a follow-up.

On Friday, December 2nd, my parents took me to Stratford and waited while I was in surgery. The surgery went well, morphine was fabulous while it lasted afterwards, and I spent the weekend recovering. By Monday, December 5th, the only discomfort I felt was the soreness from my incisions. It made it a little difficult to move about as limber as I normally would pre-pain, but I was still able to work. I honestly cannot explain my astonishment at months of constant pelvic pain suddenly disappearing completely.

My shock turned into gratification when I learned at my follow-up with Dr. Three that he did conclude I had endometriosis. He discovered endometrial tissue growing outside the uterus on my left side. I was dumbfounded though, to hear it was considered "superficial" in his opinion and was only Stage 1 (minimal). This immediately prompted me to ask why the hell I experienced *so* much pain for months, every single day.

He said, "There is no definitive reason, some people experience pain *only* during their periods and some are constant, such as yourself. That, and I've seen women with Stage 4 (severe) endometriosis not experience any pain at all and sometimes only find out about it if they're struggling with fertility and are seeking reasons why."

This blew my mind and was later proven to be very accurate. One of my best friends found out she had Stage 4 endometriosis in 2019, after trying to conceive their second child for over four years at that point. She didn't have any pain at all and already conceived one child with no struggles. It wasn't until a laparoscopic surgery was performed to clear her blocked fallopian tubes, they confirmed it was Stage 4. Not to mention the fact that a year later she had it *again* in her tubes and still didn't experience pain. I always feel such a sense of wonder, trying to wrap my head around the fact that I had Stage 1, "superficial" endometriosis, that ultimately put a halt to my daily life, and she had Stage 4, *twice*, with zero physical pain. This just goes to show how nothing is one-size-fits-all when it comes to health, and my pain was real no matter how much it was previously dismissed.

I went back to Dr. One and he recommended I stay on Visanne as a means of protecting my fertility and keeping the endometriosis at bay. At this point, the pain was non-existent, and I was living a normal life again. My month in December as a hairstylist was extremely successful and I was thankfully busy well into 2017. I had one more pelvic floor physiotherapy appointment in January after my Cuba trip, with absolutely no internal pain anymore either. My physiotherapist said my internal pain could have been my body's way of deferring pain from the developing endometriosis, like a subliminal signal something different was going on. After all that, the only worry I had was still being a player in the waiting game for my abnormal pap test.

In the spring of 2017, I had my six-month follow-up with Dr. Two which resulted in needing to schedule a cone biopsy (the removal of a cone-shaped piece of tissue from the cervix) for August 2017. My mom came with me and held my hand during the procedure and three weeks later I went back and was given the happy news of clean margins. I then had to be on a three-month biopsy schedule for a year before returning to a regular pap schedule with my family doctor. This was wonderful news to hear about my gynecological health and my state of well-being was riding the most positive wave for the rest of 2017. I was finally living pain-free, I met my current spouse in March that year, was no longer at risk from pre-cancerous cells by the end of summer, opened a salon with two friends by September (which quickly became wildly successful), and continued to see Dr. One for monitoring and future family planning.

I'd love to give all the thanks in the world to Dr. One for his dedication to his patients and their concerns. I'd also love to thank myself because I chose to fight for my body and fight to have answers despite being dismissed and feeling guilty for taking up space in hospital waiting rooms. I begged a doctor to help me and I've never felt more proud. The craziest thing about it all is if I didn't have pain that was abnormal to me, pain that forced me to hospitals, and pain that led me to beg for a second referral, I wouldn't have found Dr. One who gave me that second pap test without question and I possibly wouldn't have discovered those pre-cancerous cells. I could have been completely unmonitored for three years until my next regularly scheduled pap test with my family doctor and I can't even think about what that might have looked like. I suppose I can't say what the first gynecologist referral from my family doctor would have done for me but regardless, I don't think I could have waited that long to potentially not have that second pap test. That's devastating to wonder about.

Please don't let that devastation become something that exists in your life. Since I am a stylist, I have the absolute pleasure of befriending many women who sit in my chair and feel comfortable enough to disclose their endeavours with me. Too often, I am saddened by the number of women that have their concerns dismissed by their medical professionals, while also feeling like they shouldn't fight harder because a doctor or nurse downplayed their feelings. I am here to tell you it's okay to beg healthcare professionals. It's okay to look or feel like a lunatic and it's okay to ask for more than one referral. If you strongly believe you're in need of uncovering the truth about your health and wellbeing, then follow that belief and stand your ground. When it feels like no one cares and the healthcare system is failing you, keep digging for the one doctor that cares and be demanding about it. It will be life-altering in ways you never imagined.

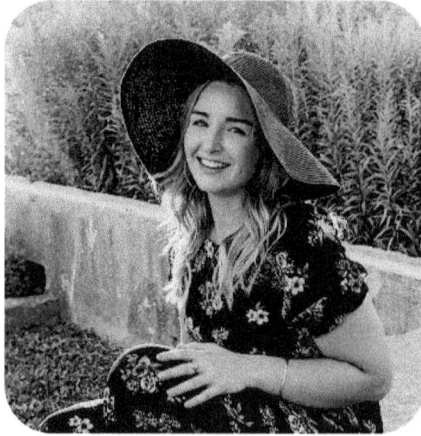

Aujha Hastings

Aujha Hastings lives in Ontario, Canada with her spouse, beautiful toddler, and two giant fur babies. She is a hairstylist and salon owner, spirit junkie, aspiring blogger and writer, and a believer of the universe. Aujha has slowly been integrating more spiritual and holistic ways of healing, in combination with modern medicine when it comes to anything she may experience when it comes to health. This can mean anything from a standard cold or ear infection to the tougher stuff requiring the expertise of doctors. Although she wishes she was aware of holistic approaches when she was diagnosed with endometriosis in 2016, all it could have done at the time is manage stress and, possibly, pain. The doctors were the cure and so was her fight and willingness to find an answer. This is her story on how she advocated for herself with doctors to find a diagnosis (quickly), what her journey gave her, and what she hopes it can give you.

IG @lotus.and.avenue | lotusavenue.org

Thank you to my family for supporting me then and now through everything. Thank you to my spouse for supporting my writing journey and the seemingly endless list of health concerns I have. Thank you to my daughter for giving me the strength I didn't even know I had. I love you all.

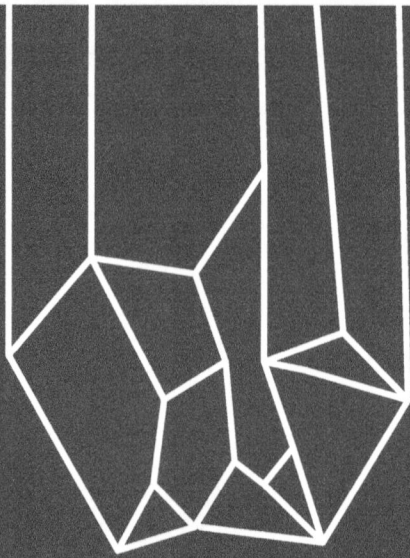

CHAPTER NINE

Misunderstood to Miss Understood

Brianna DiZeo

Anyone who knows me will tell you my family is my world and the most important value to me. Growing up, I lived in the suburbs thirty minutes from Chicago with my mom, stepdad, and brother, and would visit my biological father every other weekend. I was a bubbly kid with an old-school spirit who could be found reading a good book or writing a creative story of my own. If it wasn't either of those, I was probably at a family party or playing Sims. My love for the design of the avatars living their best life in a beautiful home kept me engaged for hours on end. I had a strong desire to be an adult and live life on my own terms, I would daydream of having a big family of my own someday to make memories to last a lifetime from Sunday dinners to spontaneous vacations to the excitement of creating our holiday traditions.

Throughout school, I was a straight-A student and enjoyed it to the fullest. School came easy to me, although I will admit fear held me back from time to time. I didn't jump for opportunity when it presented itself but watched life through the average lens. My self-worth growing

When I choose to heal, I am healing generations in my lineage.

up strictly came from the good grades I had in school. I remember getting money on holidays from uncles, aunts, or cousins of mine who were so proud of my report card. Just like most teenagers, I tried hard to fit in, and I thought good grades proved it. I felt I had to prove something to earn others' love. I thought I had to do something good for someone else to be accepted. This led to minimal healthy connections and several toxic relationships which I saw as romantic.

Don't get me wrong, I am grateful and have lived a fulfilling life but now I am ready to build towards future success more than ever before in various areas of my life. It has become clear the more I love myself and put my needs first, every aspect of my life becomes more aligned. This was not always my thought process.

Allow me to fill you in on a little bit more. My father's name is Branko and my mother's is Carmella, and yes, their personalities are as fierce as their names sound. My parents divorced when I was only a year old. Keep in mind, I was one of the only kids in my class to come from a separated family. At this time the court norm was for fathers to get every other weekend. I can count the number of times, on both hands, I have seen my mother and father in the same room, and if they were, tensions were often high, and police were often called (queue the chaos).

Nevertheless, I am extremely grateful for an amazing childhood filled with family and strong bonds but reflecting on certain childhood traumas and my personal story, allowed me to invest more into myself than ever before. I am forever grateful for my self-discovery journey and the healing that occurred along the way. When I choose to heal, I am healing generations in my lineage.

Life took a turn for the worse in my early teenage years when the court decided I could no longer see my dad. Not only did I miss out on having him present and involved regularly or for major milestones, but I also lost contact with his entire family (and we have a very large family). This was the beginning of the first of many abandonment wounds that appeared in my life. My life crumbled more than a Stella D'oro Biscuit Cookie, but I did my very best to pick up every crumb. The pain and anger remained inside me throughout the remainder of my teenage years and into early adulthood hindering my personal growth. When parents are unable to get along it becomes very uncomfortable for everyone involved and can negatively impact the child, specifically his or her emotional growth and self-worth. It wasn't until recently that I realized it was a trauma response. I couldn't clearly recall a good portion of my childhood, commonly referred to as dissociative amnesia.

My inner child often felt unsafe and unheard. I didn't belong in a courthouse or a therapist's office. My best self wasn't able to evolve while experiencing the toxic relationship my parents had. They acted negatively towards each other right in front of my innocent eyes and talked poorly of one another. I certainly know that having police intervene was only adding fuel to the fire and caused major confusion, making me feel like I was in the middle of the drama. It was a recipe for disaster making me believe that chaos was the norm and peace was foreign (especially on a major event or holiday).

For too long, I let my inner child take the driver's seat. I didn't want to lose anyone and instead of shedding my layers of trauma, I would relive my fear through one experience or another. The main issue was I led with my problems. These negative experiences were not mine to hold onto forever, but rather to pull out the life lesson and evolve.

I settled for less than I deserved.
I settled for unhealthy relationships.
I settled for average pay.
I settled for the convenient food.
I settled for living an average life.

Allow me to jump into the major construction phase of my life—my college years. Where I come from, is a small world where everyone knows everyone. I chose a college downtown in Little Italy that felt like home to me right away and coincidentally was a place my mom hung out in her late teenage years. The decision was made based on what I knew and where I felt most comfortable. It was exciting to see someone I knew as a kid or to meet people who already knew me because they were a friend of my uncle or went to grade school with my aunt. When I moved out of my house for college, I was expecting to get a degree but what I received was so much more than that—it was a whole life renovation and the beginning of my self-discovery journey.

In the beginning, however, my main focus was going out with my friends and drinking. It was the choice I made weekly as most college students do. I prioritized late nights that consisted of fishbowls (those over-the-top sugary drinks with excessive amounts of alcohol and a few fish candies) over my chemistry homework. I acted as if fun times were going out of style and even on the nights I knew I had to stay in to study, off to the club I went. How could I miss out? I spoke poorly about school and prioritized partying (my social media is proof).

Throughout my college years, not only did I accept mediocre grades, but I allowed people to walk all over me, especially those I was closest to in fear of losing them. I felt insecure with zero goals. I couldn't tell you what the next six months, three years or ten years looked like. People-pleasing was the norm, and I would overthink everything to the point of checking in with my mom or best friend before making any decision, big or small. I procrastinated a lot and spent money as quickly as I had earned it. I figured if I waited until the last minute to complete the assignment or to start studying, then I would have to accept the average grade I received. I was too scared to fail I didn't build up the momentum to get started and give it my all.

Fear of abandonment showed up constantly. The way I shook off the regret from a bad night out was to go back out the next day and do the same thing in an attempt to forget. I never understood what was holding me back until I learned all along it had been those limiting beliefs within myself and old repetitive patterns of doing what was comfortable. I settled for less than I deserved and lowered my standards far more than

I'd like to admit. I was under the impression my worth was based on the acceptance of others which was a double-edged sword when trying to build healthy relationships. The truth is, I signed a contract with fear. I was stuck in the past but didn't understand how childhood trauma and the negative implications they would hold over my belief system. I chose to live in the moment and I'm not talking about mindfulness. I failed to put myself first. I wouldn't thrive until I hit rock bottom and self-sabotage was an ongoing cycle. From procrastination to binge drinking to the point of regret and shame. I failed to put my needs first. My highest self now understands victim mode is the worst place I can be, and I don't live there. It blocks abundance and opportunities.

If it wasn't bad enough with the toxins being poured into my bloodstream from the binge drinking (which in college, we find normal) I stumbled into a toxic relationship. I remember telling my mom how great he was and she pointed out several red flags. I didn't listen and certainly learned many lessons. He was much older and offered me a sense of excitement from exploring places in the city I'd never been to. It was good until it wasn't. I was called every name under the sun but here I was continuing to be loyal and put in effort anywhere I could to make it right. I continued to wear those rose-coloured glasses and prayed for the future I dreamed of as a kid. I tried to help my then-boyfriend who wasn't willing to help himself. In doing so, I lost myself and this is never okay. I acted as if everything was rainbows and butterflies when it was far from it. I didn't share much of the dark details with family or friends until it was time to pack my belongings. I remember going to sleep one night without eating dinner. This is the moment I knew I couldn't continue. Finally, after many tears and heartbreak, I moved in silence to get out safely.

Anytime life was grand, I was hesitant to enjoy it because my mind was wondering what could go wrong next? Living in survival mode was all I knew even before I fully understood the cycle and the reasoning behind what caused it. My inner child was crying out for help and generational curses were repeating through my negative thoughts, limiting beliefs, and poor decisions. Once I became self-aware of how to build a stronger mindset my world forever changed. There is no doubt in my mind I have many who love me, but it wasn't until I recognized my worth I began to build stronger, healthier connections with everyone in my life.

My self-worth sparked once again several years later when I called off my engagement. I was briefly engaged to my daughter's father, clearly, we took steps out of order, but one month before the wedding I passed the ring across the table after too many talks. I expected more of a conversation and remembered wanting to say more but what I received was only a few words back and I knew that my intuition was right all along.

I admitted to myself this wasn't my fairytale ending.

I took off the rose-coloured glasses.

I didn't settle for less than I deserve.

I stopped taking criticism personally from people who weren't willing to help themselves.

I gave back problems that weren't mine to face.

I followed my intuition and acted on it in my best interests and my daughter's.

I took my power back.

This was the first time I had learned the true life lesson of going with the flow. What is meant to be will stay and not everyone is supposed to be in your life forever, some just a season.

That massively constructed house I had built as a kid in the Sims game wasn't built in a day. Construction goes through permit and zoning phases; we go through times where we need to heal and discover our power. To fly, I had to let go of anything weighing me down (specifically negative emotions and limiting beliefs). It took years of mistakes to realize my true inner strength. I now see the beauty in the lessons all because they led me to my healing journey and awakening that makes me my highest self: a better woman, a loving mother, a loyal partner, a caring family member, a kind friend, and a dedicated colleague. No matter what hat I am wearing, I am ready to show up fully.

I stopped taking the blame and holding onto others' baggage. I forgave myself for accepting far less than I deserve. The worry became less about how much time was wasted and a positive shift took place, which was how the lesson built the foundation for the strong woman I am today. I no longer hoped for change or played a victim in any of my circumstances. I owned my stories and the mess of each one and embraced the lesson knowing I was destined for more!

I forgave myself for accepting less than I deserved while living in survival mode. I began wanting the very best for myself and established those values. Checking in with myself frequently to ensure I was meeting my needs and to be able to take care of everything else to my full potential. From there, I began taking daily action that fulfilled me. I rewrote my story and found my power to release any thoughts holding me in that victim mentality. I now focus on what is best for me and how my future will look for my family. The biggest success is I continually create healthy boundaries and cut ties with anyone who drains my energy.

I was now focused on improving myself and determined to discover what was holding me back. Now was my time to rebuild my life from the ground up like a new construction project! Demolish what wasn't mine to hold and bulldoze through any childhood trauma that no longer served me and let go of anything and anyone who wasn't supporting me to be my highest self. Restructure *me* for who I was meant to become and live out life doing what I deserved most. Becoming who you are is truly meant to be the most liberating experience in your lifetime.

This type of shadow work was not easy, and I do take great pride in my strength for allowing the dark truths to come out to turn pain into power. The key technique that has been useful in reprogramming my thoughts is Eye Movement Desensitization and Reprocessing (EMDR) which is effective with re-writing prior experiences that may cause negative emotions or behaviours in adult life due to traumatic experiences that took place during childhood. During these sessions, I realized how little I could remember from childhood as a result of the chaos taking place around me. Throughout my EMDR sessions, I have discovered many limiting beliefs and have been able to flip the script to plan for an abundant future filled with joy and purpose. I let go of control and the outcome. Breathing in peace, exhaling negativity.

As much as we always try to rewrite the past, setting intentions and planning for the future is what I find most valuable to get to the next level in any aspect of life. My healing journey began when I decided to put myself first, signing my self-love contract. I read about personal development and listened to podcasts on my commute to work. I enrolled in courses where I enjoyed learning about holistic lifestyle approaches that bring joy and purpose to life and found inspiration more than ever before.

Losing myself was an exhausting experience. What I learned was how to pick up the pieces I needed to come back stronger. What you once knew or trusted goes out the window. The blessing is in the ability to grow back better and stronger. If you knew the reward was greater each time, would you stop at the first token? Appreciate the self-discovery journey by honouring yourself, even your past mistakes. I have proven to myself time and again I can dig myself out from the dirt, but finally, there was a shift in perspective when I realized I didn't have to get as dirty anymore. This was the key that unlocked true freedom and joy for me.

I now understand what I deserve because I am clear on my values and enforce boundaries. I understand if someone is draining my energy or I do not feel safe, I can use my voice and make the best decision. I trust myself and I love myself deeply—at my best and my worst.

I deserve to achieve my highest dreams and desires.

I deserve healthy connections and a loving soulmate.

I deserve abundance.

I deserve optimal nutrition and to fill my body with whole foods.

I deserve each and every opportunity that is on its way.

There is something remarkable about becoming a mother for the very first time. I fulfilled a childhood dream the day I became a mom, and it brings me great joy daily. Stepping into motherhood has been my biggest blessing. Having a beautiful daughter allows me to pause and enjoy the precious milestones and live in the moment daily. I embrace her high-energy personality and fun spirit as she gives her all in everything she does. It was an eye-opening experience to realize we don't choose to procrastinate or develop bad habits, but rather it is all funnelled through either negative thoughts or limiting beliefs. Raising my daughter has added tremendously to my growth journey as I'm always the one she is admiring the most.

I am proud of the woman I am professionally and also to be financially independent and have been providing for myself since my early college years. I love the *new me* who is up for challenges, and I am ready to take action towards my short and long-term goals, whereas ten years ago, I would have never even written down a goal. This ultimately translates into co-parenting with ease and doing what is in the best interests of the child. Clear evidence of breaking generational curses!

Becoming a mother has led me back to my authentic self and I love to keep evolving. Major shifts have happened especially when I decided to stop taking everything personally. I gave up trying to control situations and realized it's impossible to know every outcome. I can make friends and lose them (no hard feelings). I know, without a doubt, that I am deserving of healthy and loving relationships. I am comfortable enough to let faith lead and have trust in the outcome. And the most exciting breakthrough of all—I am proud to say I have a relationship with my father and I was the one who took initiative to reach out first, which filled a huge void I had for far too long. We can talk daily, celebrate holidays and most importantly, he can actively build a relationship with his granddaughter. I know he sees so much of me as a little girl within Daniela. For how far I've come, any setback was minor and I'm ready for what is next.

I express gratitude daily as I show up as my best self. I honour myself by knowing what I deserve and challenging myself to achieve more. Truly being my authentic self is often going back to what I enjoyed doing most as a child. My career is in the real estate field and in my free time I relax while colouring or reading. Joy to me is quality family time, especially being with my daughter. I am looking forward to all of the future vacations and holiday traditions we will make, and I love cooking family dinner on Sundays. Being my true self sparks my soul and when I'm in alignment, I can reach successful milestones and goals timely because I'm eager to check off the next box. I look forward to that sense of fulfillment when I know I gave it my all and this is where the momentum builds up to strive for even more. If life has taught me anything, it is that we get to choose to evolve or choose to repeat. Which path will you take?

Xo - Bree

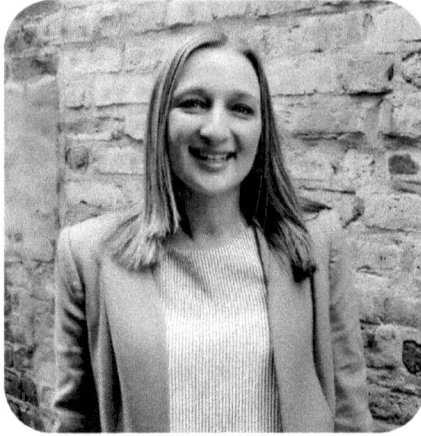

Brianna DiZeo

Brianna DiZeo grew up in the south suburbs of Illinois with a strong upbringing from Cicero where family always comes first. Brianna is a graduate of Roosevelt University with a focus on psychology and criminal justice. She later went on to receive a paralegal studies certification. Brianna chose to take a step outside of her comfort zone and explore new avenues as she welcomes a challenge. Currently, her day job is a dream come true opportunity as she has the pleasure of working with real estate investors in the lending/finance world. Inspired to show up as a dedicated and hardworking mother, Brianna knew it was her responsibility to build the life she always dreamed of. In 2020 when the world slowed down, Brianna enrolled at the Integrative Institute of Nutrition where she found her true passion in the holistic wellness space. Brianna is on a mission to support as many families as possible to be able to thrive especially with achieving optimal health. When she's not working or inspiring healthy living,

Brianna can be found spending quality time with her daughter (Daniela), enjoying a good baseball game (pending season approval), or exploring nature.

IG @breedizeo

To my younger self,

may you always recognize your worth and step into your

power as your highest self to live a life filled with peace and joy

xo, Bree

CHAPTER TEN

Seeds of Discovery

Tammy Adams

Our minds are programs running around in the background, assessing and processing the world around us. How can we relate and navigate the people that live here? My programs have a few glitches, but I am working hard to rewrite the inner dialogue that no longer serves me. There are so many things I have learned along the way I once thought I needed to survive but realize now, I need to unlearn.

As I lay here and surrender to whatever emotions come up, I can feel myself starting to breathe again. The breath goes deep into my core and my muscles begin to relax. For the past couple of days, I had been holding my breath constantly, causing pain on the right side of my stomach. It had increased so much that it forced me to use my heating pad to calm it down. This happens often when I try to avoid things. I have never looked at emotions as my friend. They were always so scary and deep. I would drown in them if I ever *really* let them in. They had to be hidden. I had to be hidden.

As a young teen, at one of my first parties with alcohol and drugs, I learned a friend of mine was cutting herself. She would take the cap of a beer bottle, squeeze it together, and use the sharp edge to draw on her skin. Why on earth did this seem like a good idea to me? I was so lost and confused about who I was and didn't think I deserved to live, while not wanting to either. This was perfect. I could regain some control. The emotions that were trying to come in could be kept away if I used this. The first time I tried it I was thirteen years old. It was like turning on a light switch.

When the flood of emotions was too strong for me to avoid, I would break apart a used razor blade, clean it off and slice the palms of my hands, my upper shoulders, or my thighs. Anywhere I could hide it from others but still have quick access to make myself hurt again. What caused me to hate myself so much? I'm sure it was a combination of things. For one, I had been sexually abused multiple times throughout my life already. This created so much shame within me, I was sure I would feel forever broken. I also didn't have a father, but no big deal right? For years I did not equate this to holding any effect on my life whatsoever. Turns out, not having my dad be a part of my life had a profound effect in shaping who I was. However, I wouldn't discover this until later on in my journey.

I tried to lock myself up and throw away the key. I did it in small subtle ways. Not speaking my mind whenever I disagreed. Apologizing, just to keep the peace, even when I felt I was right about something. Immersing myself in video games, movies and tv shows. Stealing and eating food to numb away emotions. I always felt I was not as good as everyone else around me, that there was something drastically wrong with me. In truth? It is still something I battle with to this day, just not as often, nor with the same depth.

The inner critic speaks up and says, "Who do you think you are? Nothing you have to say is important, you are wasting everyone's time." The scared inner child speaks up and says, "What are you doing? It's not safe to be seen!" A constant internal battle. Yet here I am, forty-six years old, writing a chapter in this book. Excuse me, what? I am learning more and more to live life to the fullest and follow the inner nudges of intuition, those quiet whispers from Creator, deep within my heart. Plus, I was losing sleep by not following through!

I struggled with thoughts of, how I could do this? The level of vulnerability it would require choosing to be seen by literally anyone who decided to pick up this book is slightly intimidating. And what would I write about? Who would even care? What would people think if they really saw me? This people-pleasing programming has been with me most of my life. It has always been one of the many ways I hid. It was so much easier this way.

When I was seventeen, I found

It's like the drum was watering a seed that had been planted into my DNA.

myself at an event where a First Nations band called *Broken Walls* was playing. The beat of the drum echoed deep within my heart in a way no music had ever felt before. Something was awakened in the very cells of my body. Everything else around me faded away. It's like the drum was watering a seed that had been planted into my DNA. It would be another four years before I would begin the process of understanding why but this was a pivotal turning point in my life and with my story.

As I sit here thinking about what to write, I think about my dad. How to make my dad's story connected to *my* body story? Even at this moment, I begin to feel physical pain creep up into my chest and my heart begins to race. I think I'll open the letters he wrote me. I have not read them in forever. I have talked about this so many times, with many people, but rarely have I allowed the emotions of it to rise or to be felt. I have been afraid to face it. To face her, the little girl within me that just wanted her daddy's love. What did she feel? What did she see? What did she learn? Sometimes it feels like there are more questions than answers, but when I quiet the noise around me the answers seem to trickle in more easily.

It wasn't until my early twenties while living alone in Picton, ON, that I began to wonder more and more about my dad. Who was he? Was he still alive? Did he want me in his life? If so, why had I never met him before? Do I have any other brothers or sisters? What would it be like to have them in my life? I didn't know what I would find out, but I had to do it.

I began calling directory assistance. I think the operator took pity on me because she gave me every single number listed in the small town of

Killarney with the last name Tyson. I sat and stared at the list thinking, one of these numbers could directly connect me with my father. What a strange feeling. I called the first number on the list and on that very first try someone who knew my dad answered the call. Not only that, it turned out they knew my grandmother (my father's mom, Ursula Grzelak) whom I had never met either! What are the odds? They provided me with the phone number I needed, and I hung up with disbelief. This felt incredibly surreal.

Because I felt extremely nervous to call, I decided to reach out to a friend and ask for some help. She offered to call my newly discovered grandmother while I sat beside the telephone with her. She dialled the number and I held my breath. In no time at all, they were immersed in a beautiful conversation and my body was buzzing! Suddenly my friend says, "Well she is sitting right here, do you want to talk to her?" I instantly shook my head no, but the phone was thrust into my hand. It happened so fast yet it felt like slow motion. I said "Hello?" and the first thing my grandma said to me was, "What? Did you think I would be a grumpy old grandmother?" I laughed and we continued to talk for a while. I don't remember most of what we said, but I do remember how it made me feel. I had hoped maybe I would have the other side of my family in my life, that maybe I did have a dad who loved me after all.

Grandma and I wrote several letters back and forth to each other at first. I shared copies of all of my public school photos. We decided she would tell my dad about me herself and she did. In a phone call, she told me about the letter she sent him and added she did not include any pictures of me to make him more curious to respond to her. She was such a smart woman! I wish I had had more time with her, although I am thankful for the time we did share.

In the first phone call with my dad, he alluded to the fact he did not know about me. He said when he first found out about me he was angry with my mother, but considering the circumstances of life back then, he understood. He also told me in that conversation, "Ya so ahhh, I'm native eh!" Spoken in the best Native accent ever! I will never forget how that made me feel. I was proud and it made other things seem more clear. We had a few more phone calls, but letters became our preferred form of communication.

When it came time to finally meet in person he was staying with his mom in Killarney for the winter. I arranged that I would drive up and back on the same day. I had no idea how I would be feeling, so I asked a good friend to come with me, in case I needed her to drive. It felt safe to have her with me and I am thankful for her support that day.

Along the way we noticed a man on the side of the road, it looked to me like he was hunting out of his car. Which, I didn't think was legal, so I honked the horn and waved as we went by (to help the deer escape). It was a great distraction from how nervous I was.

To my surprise, as we pulled into the driveway at my grandma's house, my dad ran to my car door and had it opened for me before I could even take my seatbelt off. There he was, excited to meet me and not hiding it one bit! (There are those tears in my eyes again). It felt so good to be loved by the person that was supposed to raise me but had never known I existed. This was the start of getting to know him and beginning to learn more about myself. We went inside and ate spaghetti my grandmother prepared. This was also the first time I had met *her* in person as well. What an emotional day. Afterwards, dad took us out to some of the places in town that were special to him. First up, was the lighthouse, where he often spent many mornings admiring the sunrise. This location would remain the most precious place in my memory, and the only picture that was ever taken with him and me together.

He proceeded to introduce me to some of his friends in town. We went to a hotel, the restaurant within it. I met a lot of people there. The only one I remember meeting was kind of embarrassing. He pointed out what kind of car I drove and said he saw me as I was driving into town. It was the same guy that may or may not have been hunting! Of course, my dad knew him, it was a small town after all. Finally, we returned to his home and spent the remainder of the evening chatting and laughing as if we had known each other forever. I noticed pictures of his other children on the wall. They had even slipped one of my school pictures underneath one of the frames. It felt so amazing and my heart was full showing me the evidence I was accepted. He talked about wanting to get us kids all together that summer to meet in person. I wanted to meet my siblings as well.

I had many questions, some I didn't even know were there, but I was still too shy to ask at the time. After all, I had a lifetime to get to know him and to find out all the answers. My friend wasn't shy though! She asked him, "So how many children do you have?" And before my dad could answer my grandma put her hand on his shoulder and said, "Five, that we know of." My dad laughed and said he had been a little wild in his youth.

Life was not easy for my dad, however, the day we spent together was evidence he had joy in his heart and a great sense of humour. He talked about when he was a tour guide and when he would convince the tourists the white quartz rock way up high in Killarney Park was snow! I could picture him in the boat telling them as though it was one of the other facts he was to share with them.

Here are some things my Dad said to me in the first letter he ever wrote me.

"You are a very pleasant surprise and I'm looking forward to meeting you sometime soon."

"I wish you could spend some time here with me."

"Right now I wish I could give you a big hug and tell you I love you and I'm sorry I wasn't there when you were growing up. I do love you Tammy and look forward to seeing you."

"You are very pretty in your pictures"

He was full of compliments and always wrote how he felt. I will always be grateful that he did.

When they say "you are not promised tomorrow so make the most of today" it is true. I can't think of a single regret from the times I was brave and did the hard thing but I will forever regret not jumping in and spending more time with my dad and my grandma before they passed away. I thought I would have the rest of my life to get to know him. This will always be one of my biggest regrets.

I remember the day I found out that my dad had passed away. I had been away on a canoe trip with a friend, working as a leader for her Out-Tripping company with youth. I had missed his funeral as the trip was days long and there was no way of communication with us out on the water. It was such a shock to my system and a lot to process. How do you grieve the loss of someone that should have been close to you, but you didn't even get the chance to know? How do you grieve not just the loss of all of the previous years you missed out on, but the loss of any possible moments in the future? Moments of talking about everything or nothing at all. Moments of making memories to cherish forever.

His leaving my life so soon after finding him was also the loss of meeting my siblings (three sisters and a brother). The meeting dad had wanted to create was taken away and although I have made attempts to reach out to them, thus far it has been a no-go. This is a sadness that is always with me yet I also cannot be upset with them, because this whole thing has to be hard for them too. I have hope we will one day be in each other's lives.

Things I learned about my dad from one year of knowing him:
1. He loved me.
2. He loved his mother.
3. He loved his other daughters and son.
4. He had regrets in his life but he was attempting to live in the moment.

5.   He loved to fish.

6.   He loved the outdoors.

7.   He was an early riser.

8.   He did not like writing letters but did so anyway because he wanted to get to know me.

9.   He was a handyman, able to fix things even in remote places.

10. He liked to take pictures.

11. He wanted to spend time with me.

12. He was Native. Ojibway (Anishinaabe).

13. He went to powwows.

14. He loved dogs.

15. He loved hiking.

16. His handwriting was better than mine!

Uncovering my roots of being Anishinaabe (Ojibway) has had such a positive impact on my heart. A way of getting to know my dad even though he was gone. It's deep, it's personal and hard to explain. Part of me does not want to talk about it because of how much my inner critic judges me. "You are not qualified to talk about this because you should have learned your language more by now," and, "you should have gone to more powwows and other native events that would help you learn more," and, "you should have invested more money into new regalia by now." I could continue, but you get the point. It's not fun to "should" on yourself. The truth is this is my life and my heart so I am the only one qualified to share the impact this has had on me.

The first time I wore regalia was at an event at a church I was attending in Belleville, ON. It was their first-ever First Nations conference. The band playing turned out to be the same band I had heard of when I was seventeen! What a coincidence! The moment I heard about this weekend event I knew in my heart I needed to attend. So much so that I rescheduled my wedding day! Now that I am no longer married, I can confidently say I made the right decision. I knew in my heart this held some significance in my life and absolutely nothing was going to keep me from attending.

This wasn't a typical Christian conference. It wasn't churchy people feeling sorry for "the poor natives" and what can we do to make ourselves feel better and teach them a better way. No. This was different. This was a Native lead conference. The music, the dancers and the speakers were all Native leaders helping and teaching people about reconciliation and our traditions. I had no idea at the time how rare this was. There are many misconceptions about believing that for one to dress in regalia and use the Native drum is evil. They taught at this event that the deer that was used to make the drum was a good deer that had never sinned. Native humour is the best humour!

When I had planned to attend this event I did not know I would be invited by some of the dancers to join them in the Grand Entry one night. A beautiful woman allowed me to borrow one of her regalia sets. They helped me get prepared in the back to come out with them and dance before our Creator. To dance for the healing of those around us. Our dance was not a show, but a prayer in motion from our hearts. Now, if you knew me back then, let's just say, dancing in public was not my thing. Dancing was always saved for behind closed doors, music blasting while cleaning my home. Alone. Please understand that to have been a part of this was a very big step outside my comfort zone. But at the moment, being asked to dance with them made my heart pound so loud I could hear it and the butterflies inside my stomach were already dancing.

Feeling such freedom in that experience is difficult to put into words. The sense of being a part of what I now know was meant for me, moving to the beat of the drum, reaching all the way to my core. And it was more than just a feeling of belonging, but that was part of it. It was a sense of being one with who I was created to be, a glimpse of the real me. The *me* that is here to dance and bring healing to the earth.

Since that first time, I have had many opportunities to join with others to dance like this. To help spread awareness and be a part of reconciliation. It feels like my very existence as a Native woman is in itself an act of defiance. As I learn more about my culture and language, I get to be a part of breaking generational trauma and giving hope to future generations.

This part of my life has not come without emotions to process, however, the more I learned about the truth of what happened to my ancestors. Massacres, residential schools, reservations being placed strategically to not thrive, treaties agreed to and never upheld, and missing and murdered Indigenous women that the police and RCMP never bother looking for. The anger grew within me as well as sadness and disgust. Feeling helpless to do anything about any of it.

I used to be proud of the fact I was Canadian but the truth about how our country came to be took that away from me. Canada Day and Thanksgiving will never feel the same. The ambivalence that happened in my heart was not easy. Wanting to forgive and move on but still unable to, I had to grieve.

We don't have to look far to see the injustices still occurring to this day. How does one grieve something that perpetually continues? One day at a time. Listening to what we need each day and a boatload of self-care and self-compassion. Allowing our emotions to flow, unapologetically. Breathing in the present. Sounds like I have it all figured out, eh? I do not.

In the meantime, I continue to learn more about the language and culture, incorporating these things into my everyday life and taking time to celebrate the small victories right now. The sheer fact that a couple of years ago or less taking up space was very uncomfortable. Even something as simple as stretching out on my yoga mat, being asked to take up space that way was impossible unless I was covered by a blanket. In my own home and alone I felt unsafe, shame came over me and the need to hide was there. Now? I can take up space with or without a blanket—shame-free. Another example was how I slept in my bed. Hugged in close to the very edge. Someone could have easily slept on the other side without even knowing I was there. I was so far away in only a double-sized bed. Now? I take my half out of the middle! Not sure how I would ever go back to being so small there. I own that space.

I am very thankful for the Native Friendship Centres that offer language lessons. They welcome everyone regardless of their cultural background. If you want to learn more you can reach out to your local friendship centre and see what programs they have that you can take part in. I remember when I first started to go to the one in Toronto. One day I showed up for class there were a few people outside and as I went past it was the first time I had heard the Ojibway language outside of class or a cultural event. I was at a loss for words and a little embarrassed. You know when someone says "hello" but they say it with an emphasis that becomes flirting? Well, that's what happened as I walked past the one guy out front. It was "Aniin." I didn't know how to respond to flirting in English, never mind Anishinaabe!

Now, where I live here in London, ON, I was able to attend a few weeks of Ojibway language classes at the local Friendship Centre, but unfortunately all in-person sessions were shut down due to covid. This was very discouraging, but I also found other resources online to continue to learn more. Tribal Trade offers Indigenous Teachings, workshops and has smudge kits and other items for sale. I was able to take one of their online courses at a time when I needed to have a better focus in life.

When I was invited to a photoshoot with authors in this book project, it felt like I was getting ready for ceremony. Ceremony feels sacred. Not just for special occasions as I was once programmed to believe. Life itself is sacred and all the intricate pieces of it. The day-to-day otherwise mundane aspects of life can be filled with intention, grace and determination. Inviting Creator to be a part of each moment can make every day a ceremony of life. I feel the difference in my heart. When I have slipped into the doldrums of life, living in a way of avoidance and hiding or when I show up, wide awake and ready to feel all the feels of the day and be seen for who I am now and not the Tammy of yesterday.

Today's Tammy loves herself, puts herself first knowing that if I don't fill my own cup I have nothing to give to other people. I know now that life is a process that never ends and there is no finish line. There is always more to learn and unlearn and it does not have to feel impossible. When I give myself space to feel without judgment in the midst of all of the lessons it can go so much easier. Something that would have been impossible for me at one time but I am a different person now. The programs running in the background of my mind have changed so much I often find myself thinking, *who am I?* But in a *good* way, as I am so very proud of all of the progress I have made.

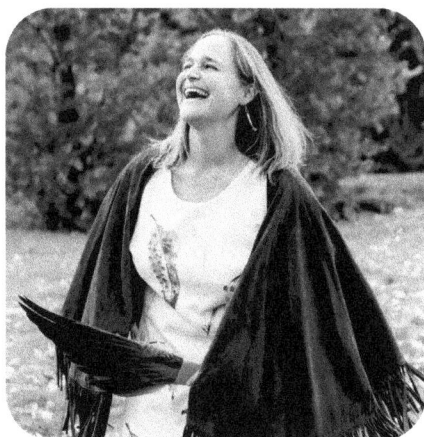

Tammy Adams

Tammy Adams was born and raised in Northern Ontario where her love for the outdoors first began. She now lives in London, Ontario where she is a letter carrier and gets to spend most of her days outside. On her days off, you can find her hiking long trails, being captivated by the beauty that surrounds her. Tammy has been passionate about inner healing and self-development forever. Through her lived experiences, her infectious laugh and her loving personality, Tammy is a treasured friend to so many. Having learnt of her native roots, Tammy is dedicated to learning all she can about her heritage. Tammy continues to be a light in every room she walks in and loves to laugh with others.

IG @anishinaabewoman

I would like to give a special thank you to Kim Basler who helped me love myself at a depth I never thought possible. Without your questions I both loved and sometimes hated, I am sure I would at best, still be attached to my couch in depression and at worst, I would have left this earth already. Thank you Kim for believing in me until I could find that belief for myself also!

CHAPTER ELEVEN

The Dance Within Me

Patrice Burns

The heart is a place of deep excavation and ayahuasca helped me dig. If you are not familiar with this beautiful spirit, she is the grandmother of plant medicine and she will show you what you need to see to find a path of where you need to go. In short, this is what you came here to discover. The discovery of *you* is the most important work you'll ever do.

Ayahuasca started with a whisper until finally, she got me on the mat. Plant medicine changed my life by magnifying the connection between my head, heart and stomach. Not only is the heart anatomically structured above the stomach, but it also lives within the diaphragm more often than not. My body has been a blueprint and the greatest gift to unwrap. I spent the first five to six years of my life unable to talk and this is where I would learn what humiliation felt like. I would be the girl no one wanted to listen to or have patience for. This would be the introduction to a life where it seemed I didn't belong and where I felt unseen, ignored and misunderstood, more often than not.

Throughout my teenage years, I was in and out of hospitals. Times where I played games of holding my breath until I passed out, to when I was hit so hard with a soccer ball at the age of fourteen. The soccer ball injury was an important one though, as it led to a discovery I might not have otherwise found—a tumour in my right breast. What I realize now is the emotional heartache I was experiencing during this time and the shame for causing grief to my parents. From that crazy game in the schoolyard when my parents were breaking up, to the tumour found a year later when my parents were getting back together. A direct correlation for sure.

Heartbreakingly, after the surgery to remove the tumour my father suddenly passed away. This would be when I put my armour on, which would lock away the little girl inside for decades to come. My younger self, the one who held my pain would not be seen again until my introduction to ayahuasca.

In the first year of high school, after the tumour was removed and my father passed away, my body battled something fierce. This was supposed to be the biggest year of a young teen's life, but for me, my body, mind and soul were suffering. I was pencil thin back then and finally becoming a woman but now one of my breasts had been ripped open. For as long as I could remember all of the ailments I endured throughout my teenage years, brought me back to either not feeling loved, not being enough, or feeling humiliated. Losing the sensation in my right breast turned out to be the inability to breastfeed my children and a shaming I held onto for years.

Within weeks of my father dying I would get my first period, my hormones were raging, and my body felt like it was failing. I couldn't go a day without sweat pouring out of me as the emotional uprisings I brought up daily were mounting. What was happening? Here I go, back to the hospital again, this time learning I suffered from an overactive thyroid, and it needed to be removed. Another surgery. This resulted in medications for life. With blood tests given regularly and the prescription altered often, no wonder my body struggled to stay functional. Humiliation became a daily struggle for me as my family would start to tell me to go take a pill whenever I was emotional. How could they possibly understand how it felt to be me?

Despite all of this, I knew my heart was aching as I fought to belong and to keep up. I survived the death of an abusive alcoholic father and a widowed mom with three out of five kids still living at home. I made it through those teenage years as best as I could. It is through the ugliest parts of my childhood I learned of the spaces that needed healing and my body helped me find them.

When I say I survived I didn't mean I came out whole. At eighteen years old I required a tonsillectomy which would be the surgery that changed my life forever. My journey comes from a view with my own spirituality and what has brought me to who I am today. I have been the girl who looked for signs my entire life or looked at things from a different perspective, all the while hiding my internal light and many times being questioned for it.

My tonsillectomy would soon become a lifetime sentence from a botched surgery by way of an accidental removal of my uvula due to a slip of the hand, a mistake. Many would ask what a uvula is but not if you are ever-present for my "goose laugh." Losing my uvula had me landing in emergency rooms when food would go up instead of down. Without my uvula, *the choke gland*, which I would soon know it by, turned out to be a hazard for my well-being. For years I would experience liquid pouring out of my nose even though I ingested it through my mouth. To this day I dread being sick as it doesn't feel good coming out of my nose.

If you are one of my kids, you were either entertained or resentful of this laugh. When I have that most perfect belly laugh the goose comes calling and the choking erupts. I remember being on a pirate ship ride once when my laughter started. My goose call arrived as my panic set in and the conductor stopped the ride to let me off. One of my kids got stuck on that ride and I am still unsure if this is one of their childhood wounds. For me, the fear of choking to death by way of laughter is real because I suffer from nervous laughter. The rule at our house with the kids is if I start laughing uncontrollably and my hands go to my throat, call 911. I cannot count the number of times heads have turned with people thinking, "What in the hell is that?" Don't worry, it's just me— laughing and choking to death.

In 2010, I had the fortune or misfortune to tame my goose laugh and to this day I wish I had it back. I wanted to go zip lining but was afraid to die hanging upside down in the jungle laughing when a gentleman approached introducing me to EFT (Emotional Free- dom Technique). This stranger would soon become a friend after sharing a gift that has helped me to this day. He took me to the side and started explaining how I was to follow all of his tapping points on my face with my fingertips just as he was doing, repeating his words. After a fifteen-minute tapping session, I was sent on my way to face a

Laugh often, as it's healing for the soul.

fear I could not have imagined doing before this. I made it up to the jungle canopy, zip-lined to my heart's content and upon exiting the jungle turned to him and said, "Give me back my laughter." Because of this experience, my belly laughs rarely surface and the nervous laughter is just a belly ache. I never thought I would say I miss the fear of choking by way of laughter because the truth is we all love a good belly laugh. I am however confident there will come another day when the goose appears and I might be triggered by responses once again.

The lesson I want to take from this experience specifically is to *not let your faults or traumas get in the way of your celebrations*. This is your story and you are meant to tell it. Laugh often, as it's healing for the soul. Remember that laughter is not always present so try to embrace the lighter moments instead of holding onto the trauma you may have.

Throughout the chapters of my life, I would discover our Chakra Energy System and how I could heal through energy work. I learned I could heal my body, my mind and my heart—my spirit. This explained so much to me and many began rolling their eyes bringing me back to those feelings of humiliation. In truth, I was a girl who shrank in fear of being ridiculed or worse not being seen. I controlled the fear of sharing pain and frustration, only to share my tears which slowly felt out of control.

My tears were the cesspool of my entire existence it seemed. All my emotions have come through with tears, whether it is anger, heartbreak, humiliation, or a simple conversation that shares my inner meaning. The conflict my body suffered with was a mixture of tears trapped by the armour I put on the day I stepped out of the limousine for my father's funeral. The tears, the people in my life who chose not to see me, would one day fade away from my life.

How did all of me survive? I can only say it is because I chose to heal through my tears and eventually embrace them. My two favourite emotions are laughter through tears or tears through laughter. I had no choice but to bond with who I was if I wanted to become who I was meant to be.

My story didn't stop at my tonsillectomy because at the age of twenty I woke up to the most intense rash on my body. This rash had my family running for shelter as I was unable to function. This rash covered my body from the top of my head to the tips of my toes including the palms of my hands and the bottoms of my feet. I swelled up, unable to wear shoes or look in the mirror. The family joked about covering the mirrors and a twenty-year-old being brought to Sick Kids was so emotionally painful. Without answers, I was sent home and whatever happened to me was soon forgotten as the rash peeled off of my body like a snake's shedding of its skin.

Throughout my early years, I learned to shut my innermost self inside and to hold my breath. I have struggled my entire existence with shallow breathing or holding my breath. Was this because of a game I played at the age of twelve? I will never know. I can only understand it as me being afraid of what will come next. There was always a next and I was always struggling to breathe.

As I navigated through the next chapters of my life, I would encounter many battles within my body. By my late thirties-early forties, my body was writing its own story. The beginning would be a journey with vertigo where I was unable to move, let alone function in life as a newly divorced mother of two. Vertigo crippled me for over six months as my young children tried to understand. Soon enough this brought me back to the hospital. As they probed for answers, once again there were none. My body was giving me signs there was a pain that lay within, and my physical body was only a symptom. If vertigo did not pull me out of my emotional and spiritual pain, then my body was going to begin the work for me. I went from hip pain needing cortisone to fibromyalgia prescribing Lyrica. I spent three years with quarterly ophthalmologist visits after being told I had the onset of glaucoma.

As my mom was dying and I felt the pain of becoming an orphan, I started bleeding out with adenomyosis. What was I not seeing and why was my body asking me to look deeper? It would be so much easier if the doctors had answers to give me. My soul, my intuition was telling me there was something greater going on and I was to keep searching. I threw out the Lyrica after three days and began to search further.

I spent a lifetime being told I was a mystery more times than not, so I did my own probing and went back to school. I studied energy work and body and spiritual psychotherapy. I looked for the changes that were required of me to find a happy equilibrium in a life I did not understand or connect with. I was losing a grip on my life and my tears would eventually introduce hyperventilating to my nervous system. This was all followed by my wound of humiliation making life feel unbearable. I was embarrassed and believed it was a weakness—that was what I had learned and now must unlearn.

My tears, my emotions, and my outlet were not a weakness. This is what we are taught when others are uncomfortable with tears. How did I let myself be confused by who I was because others saw me as weak? For me, this last year has given me many great teachings as well as my greatest healing. I recognize when the feelings are coming up because my body has its own dance. My tears start to brew, my breathing shallows, hyperventilating sets in and then the most embarrassing part of me—my babbling from five years old resurfaces and I am no longer able to formulate my thoughts, let alone my words. My head begins a dialogue with my heart, my diaphragm, and my stomach—my loop (the dance) wreaks havoc on my nervous system. My stomach has been an ongoing issue and fear for me as it often can call in my vertigo. These feelings, physical or emotional are all interchangeable in my being and my body and have caused me great pain through the years.

In 2014, I would experience an emotional breakdown that would be another defining moment in my life. I was going to take my body back by enrolling in yoga teacher training. I was going to move the emotions instead of succumbing to them and I was going to learn to breathe properly. In 2015, I would learn how my heart was the driving force of my body more than I ever realized. We all know when we are hurting, our heart for some inexplicable reason hurts physically, more so than any other organ in our body. I will forever remember February 19th,

2015 when my heart was wrenching in pain. I truly believe it twisted up in my diaphragm along with my small intestine. I know the agony of this feeling came from an emotion I would never want to experience again; my heart was fully breaking. That night I realized the same pain is what I must have given my mother. The unforgiving feeling I felt for myself only compounded my pain. I would one day learn to love and finally forgive myself. This is where I learned the power and strength of my heart. This is when I began to heal.

When the invitation to plant medicine showed up in my life, many people tried to dissuade me. What I would come to realize is that if ayahuasca has a gift for you her whispers turn to screams and she shows up everywhere. This is when I knew it was time to heal. I started listening to myself and not the people who couldn't see me. Plant medicine is the gift that brings you to the fear and the doorway to what lies within. I have done many retreats, schooling, and healing over the years but what came out of my ayahuasca journey could not have been more surprising. I was amazed this plant was the experience I had been yearning for.

This past summer, ayahuasca brought me to the battlefield of my body. The first ceremony brought in the head pain with the stomach pain and I was left praying on my mat. I silently suffered through my pain while asking for the answers to my life. By the second ceremony, my vertigo took a stronghold of me and I knew I was never returning to ayahuasca. I have lived in fear of my vertigo for the past fifteen years and that is what the spirit of ayahuasca showed me.

When I was told I had to do breathwork that weekend I went into an even more excruciating pain as I couldn't even stand up, let alone do the one thing I have been fighting with my entire life (breathing). The experience left me speechless as I was able to meet my fourteen-year-old self. I connected to the day of my father's funeral where I handed my younger self an emotional armour telling her I couldn't do the pain anymore. Ayahuasca brought me full circle to a part of my soul I had locked up deep inside. My younger self carried me through life and at what cost to her I am slowly discovering. I fell in love with every part of me that day as I was shown the beauty that had been waiting inside. I was able to release the stuck energy of years gone by and in turn, I was able to release myself.

I have been learning that everything within my body is connected and I am healing one cell at a time. The last two years have given me the space to fall in love with my heart and my soul. I believe all of the shame I had been carrying was not even mine to carry.

If you were to have asked me just a few short months ago what my body was trying to tell me, I would answer that ayahuasca was not for me. Now I can honestly say ayahuasca showed me the window to my soul and once again the spiritual work brought me back to my bodywork. During the first ayahuasca ceremony, my stomach pain did not let up. I spent the summer looking for the understanding of why the constant pain. I believe your body speaks your mind and my body was telling me something *big*. I tend to lean into my understanding, but I also lean into what the medical doctors have to say. Through blood work and an endoscopic procedure that would once again provide no answers. It was time to lean into my practices and tools.

Not all of my tools will be your tools. Believing in your strengths will bring you on a path that leads you towards your discovery. My journaling, my meditation practices, my energy tools as well as my insistent belief there is a greater power within, brought me to the person I am today. I know with every fibre of my being that retreat work is a necessary evil and a gift for my continued healing. Our healing is never finished and that is the beauty you are invited to discover. No more will I hold on to the fear of the judgment of others when I decide to go to the jungle to heal. It has taken me many years to find where my soul meets heaven and for me, the jungle is where that happens.

Leaning into my practices I found past life regression therapy and through various sessions, I learned how my heart and my stomach were connected. I spent my whole life questioning why my heart was always in pain or was never held the way I knew it should be. In my past lives, I would learn not only the truth of my heart but the pain that I experienced in those lifetimes. After the second regression, I was journaling days later to realize my diaphragm and tummy were not ailing me, then I wondered. Did my going back to earlier soul lives give me the healing I have been sifting through in this lifetime? Or is it because I am finally listening to the call of my soul to write? After my regressions, I was called by my heart to write after hiding this part of me away for so long.

Today I can tell you my stomach, diaphragm and heart connection found a miracle in past life regression therapy and my therapy of writing. My practices brought me to the other side—to my joy and my heart. Our heart and soul truly do carry the answers—you just have to look inside; you have to listen.

The energy work and body psychotherapy gave me more answers

right down to the crippling of my hips that for a decade moved from one side to the other. When the pain was in my left hip I was struggling to move on from my divorce and our family trauma that ensued. The left side of our body represents our feminine energy, and I was struggling in a heartbreak I thought was larger than me. When the pain landed in my right hip (the masculine energy) I knew she was trying to slow me down as at this time, I was doing too much. My body was completely out of balance with the Yin my feminine energy and the Yang my masculine energy was fighting to function. With the help of Myofascial Release Therapy (MFR) along with learning more about our beautiful piriformis and psoas muscles (the encasing and armour) of all of our inner workings, I am on the road to understanding the dance within my body.

Leaning into the medical field and my practices I discovered a link between them both. The magical wandering nerve, our vagus nerve that connects into all of our messiness—our juiciness. We have to explore the path our vagus nerve travels. The medical doctors of today are slowly giving notice and I believe it is a big part of my story.

The vagus nerve will share my physical answers alongside the spiritual practices I carry within. I have chosen to trust in my wandering nerve and the bodywork I believe in. Upon learning the vagus nerve starts in our brain (my first injury) and runs through our thorax touching on all of our inner organs I now know this is something to explore. From a young age, I was dealing with my voice, thyroid and tonsils. As life went on I would be fighting with emotions, breathing, and stomach problems all the way down into my hips. Learning that the vagus nerve runs into the parasympathetic nervous system is all the telling I need.

Somewhere along the way, my vagus nerve got entangled and if you follow my blueprint you will see it tells my story. You can also ask if this was my story from the very beginning as I came into the first six years of my life fighting to talk. This is where my loop started—this is my dance. You see, I came into this life with a wound and I believe I am on the brink of healing it. I believe all of those mysterious ailments and surgeries were a part of my journey that led me here today. I was meant to be different, and I have spent my lifetime unwrapping my gift—my heart. The mysteries were about seeing the underlying messages and not the pain. I can honestly say I know what loving myself truly means now. I can finally see who I am and who I came here to be.

I have discovered the only person that needs to see me is ME!

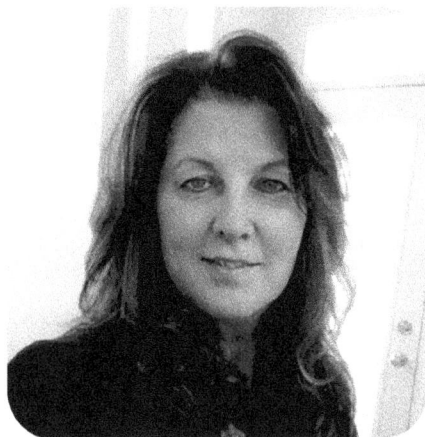

Patrice Burns

Patrice Burns is a passionate entrepreneur who hung up her real estate hat to share her journey to help guide others in theirs. Her journey of self-healing began in school at, Transformational Arts College in Toronto. At an early age, she struggled to find her place in this world. Her body would be an invitation for her to learn who she was meant to become. What she has discovered in her work is that our body speaks our mind and if we choose not to listen—spirit will trip us up. Patrice has spent almost two decades pursuing her answers to what she knew laid within. Collecting various healing modalities and pursuing some unconventional practices, Patrice found her way to heal. When it comes to heartbreak Patrice found the ability to *heal*, *love* and *forgive*—her heart has never failed her. This is why she opened up a quaint little shop in Brighton, Ontario. It is a container and an invitation for others to begin their journeys into their heart and their healing. This is why she officiates weddings, runs special events including retreats and most recently built a labyrinth. Patrice has chosen to heal her wounds and limiting beliefs. She continues to chip away at the armour she built up since childhood. She empowers and guides others to transform their wounds, their stories and to completely change their lives. Everyone has the choice to bring their heart into the light and this is where you will find hers.

IG @patricejburns | FB @patricejoanburns

www.patriceburns.com

To my wonderful children Kirstyn and Robert who stood by me through many of those dark times. I know it was not always easy and you lost a Halloween in there somewhere but I sure do love you both—**I'll love you forever, I'll like you for always, as long as I am living, my babies you'll be.** It is because of you both I continue to heal. To Spirit I am filled with gratitude—I have been surrounded and held my entire lifetime by you. You have helped me discover the blueprint of my soul and have helped me heal some pretty big wounds. It is so true—you do have our backs. Thank you to Grandmother Ayahuasca, your plant medicine helped me to discover some hidden parts that still needed to heal.

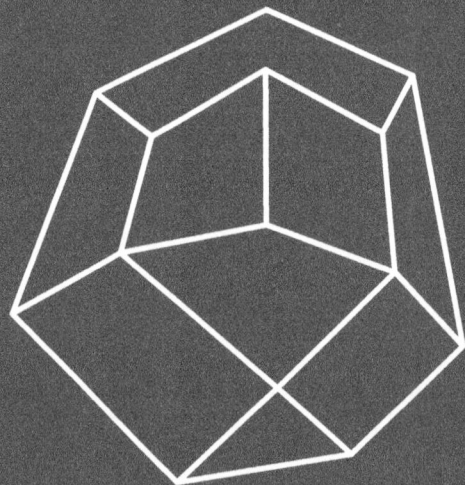

CHAPTER TWELVE

I'm Not Still Here By Accident

Amber Nicole

I stepped into the bathroom and stood in front of a mirror; only this mirror had a picture inside its frame instead of reflecting my image back to me. I looked at this picture of a girl intently for a long while. I studied her face. She looked lost and empty; like she was looking through me. Her face was pale and limp, her eyes sunken in and tired with black circles underneath them, and her mouth lay still and emotionless. There was nothing to this girl. Whatever her character used to be, her personality, her looks—it had been stripped from her. What happened to her? I studied this picture over and over and as I looked once more, I saw the picture blink. That's the moment I realized there was no picture. The girl in the frame was me. The sad, lost, empty, emotionless girl staring back at me was me. How had I gotten to this point? Was there nothing left of me? Was I that far gone? Was there no hope left?

★ ★ ★

I sat at the glass kitchen table as I waited for her to show up. I felt nervous and afraid of what she would say to me. Did I really need her in my life? My gaze held the floor for dear life as my arms crossed my stomach in preparation to have to talk about some difficult things. My mom greeted her at the door and led her into the house to meet me. She exuded confidence and care in the way she walked and the expression her face held. Here I am, sitting at this table, living at my mom's house for a whole two days, my kids at school and daycare as I try to digest everything that has just gone on and accept help. I was referred to Women's Crisis Services and that's who walked into my mom's home. She asked me a bunch of questions about what happened, how I got here and filled out the necessary paperwork. I was vacant, had no affect, refused to make eye contact, and instead held my gaze on the floor and did not remove my arms from their protective resting place, folded across my abdomen. I answered all her questions with no emotional response, no inflection to my words. I was flat, I felt utterly deflated. I minimized everything that happened and claimed it wasn't as bad as her fancy checklist proved it was. I didn't trust her. What did she know anyway? For all she knew, I was making it up. She told me I had just left a horrendously abusive marriage and I was still in danger.

✷ ✷ ✷

I was involved in an abusive marriage for six years. I was married at age twenty. I was feeling desperate for love and affection after a sexual assault left me feeling raw when I was seventeen. I wanted what other people had. I wanted their happiness, their zest for life, their dreams and aspirations. I wanted to be just like all of the happy people out there but instead, I was battling the war within my mind. That war kept me in silent turmoil for years, hell, it still keeps me silent sometimes. This part of my journey is not over but when I step back into the places that robbed me of everything, I find those were the experiences that shaped the person I am now. The circumstances I was dealt in life only helped to create the tenacious woman I am now.

I became pregnant just two months after I was married and I did not appreciate that test result. I was in college and I was only twenty years old. I did not want to be pregnant. I did not want to be a mom. My emotions flew all over the place during that pregnancy. I contemplated giving the baby up for adoption, I knew I was in a bad place, and I was not going to be safe there with a baby to take care of too. The war in my mind escalated to a new level of intensity and I feel like I broke when I was six months pregnant. It was starting to become obvious I was pregnant, and I knew I had hit a point of no return. I felt trapped and terrified.

∗ ∗ ∗

One more damn fight. I felt so awful about myself. I was such a burden, a selfish bitch. I grabbed my keys and headed out the door. I had a bridal shower to go to. Sitting in the car I started to lose control of my emotions. I kept looking at my phone while I drove, reading countless text messages. I didn't respond. This is enough, I'm not doing it anymore. I need to get out of here, I need to protect us. I started driving frantically, speeding on the highway, changing lanes erratically. I felt out of control. I was crying uncontrollably and apologizing to my belly. To my son. I took my seat belt off when I reached 150km/h. I drove, feeling the adrenaline pump through my blood, black pupils taking over any bit of colour in my eyes. I put my seatbelt back on and slowed down. I took the next exit off the highway and pulled over. Crying uncontrollably still, I put my head in my hands and screamed. This was not going to be my life. I started driving again, crying, with the same intensity. This time when I drove, I had a mission. I entered back onto the highway and started driving quickly again. Heart pulsing, hands sweaty and shaking, I saw my opportunity. I veered off the road and drove right into a hydro pole. Crash. Metal crunched and glass shattered across the grass; airbags blew up and shoved my chest back into the driver's seat. The car flipped and landed on the driver's side. I opened my eyes. "Fuck." I thought. It didn't work. "Did I just kill my baby?" I thought, struck by fear, a paralyzing, almost inconceivable fear. I climbed out of my car and was helped down to the grass by a man. He walked me over to the curb to sit down. I was holding my belly, apologizing, asking him to please stay alive. I wouldn't hurt him again. I promised. After a few hours in the emergency room, I stopped having contractions and I was told that my son was going to be okay. I was lucky. We were both lucky. A nurse looked at me with care flooding through her eyes as she asked me what happened. When I tried to tell her I'd just been so tired of being pregnant and I fell asleep at the wheel I was choked by tears. The tears slid down the sides of my face as I lay on a hospital bed still clutching my belly. The nurse asked me if it was really an accident and I broke into a convulsing, panicked cry. She put her hand on my head and stroked my hair. She was going to help me.

The journey continued to escalate over the years. I felt defeated, trapped, alone and horrendously depressed. I had no hope left in my life. My decision-making was impulsive and irrational and I just needed to survive a little longer, yet my will to do so kept dwindling. Four years after my son was born, I gave birth to my second son. I thought, *having another baby will surely make things better*—wrong. So very wrong. Living in the situation I was living in, feeling the emotions I was feeling, or not feeling, and hiding behind a fake smile and made-up happy stories is not the place nor the life for another child. I was desperate. I needed things to get better. My life was far from what I wanted it to be but I started to accept there was nothing better outside of my life. I was stuck. When I was pregnant the second time, I started to lose hope even more. The abuse continued throughout the pregnancy and I didn't fight back. I didn't care anymore. I didn't care about myself. At about five and a half months pregnant I lost a family friend to suicide. The grief I felt at that time was insurmountable, devastating. I knew how close I'd been to suicide before and how terrifying it was and to find out someone I grew up with had died by suicide was too much to take in. My hormones were all over the place, coupled with all the emotions I'd been experiencing for years and it was too much. Too much grief. I don't remember much of the end of my pregnancy, but I certainly remember the delivery.

✷ ✷ ✷

Congratulations, Amber! He's perfect! The doctor and nurses said to me as I finished pushing my son out of me. We will wash him up and bring him to you. Emotionless I lay on the hospital bed sweating, in lots of pain, exhausted, waiting for my son to be brought over to me. This perfect baby. "Here he is!" The nurse exclaimed walking over to me with the son I should have never had. If it wasn't socially unacceptable, I think I would have denied this offer. I did not want my son. No, please don't make me bring him home to this life. He deserves so much more than what he will get living with me. I don't want him. I took the baby in my arms and felt no joy; instead, I felt guilt in every cell in my body.

Postpartum depression is real. It's often not talked about in detail yet it's something so common it's pathetic there's not more information and support for it. I felt such intense distaste for this little baby. He was adorable and precious and innocent, but I didn't love him. I didn't want him. I was followed by a midwife for the first six weeks after his birth and she was the one who called a psychiatrist for me after I went into her office two weeks postpartum and cried the entire time. I didn't tell her how bad it was getting but she knew I was not well. In hindsight, that psychiatrist referral saved my life. Five months into postpartum, my mood hit an all-time low. I hated my life. I hated being a mom, I hated being a wife, I hated being alive. The guilt that was consuming any shred of hope became so overwhelming and ever-present I had to take action. I rationally thought that if I took the lives of myself and my baby I would be saving myself and my son from the world I desperately hated and didn't trust. However, the irrational part is the murder-suicide it would take to complete the action felt like the only way to freedom. To say this time in my life was dark is an understatement. No words can describe the depth of my despair, the overwhelming, unyielding guilt and anger I was living with every day; I wanted out. I needed out. And so I made a plan.

It was a Monday when I came up with a plan on how to take my life. I had the method, the location, the date and the time all figured out. I would go to bed on Friday night, and be awoken by an alarm at 2:00 am with instructions to kill myself. I had an appointment with the psychiatrist on Wednesday and I just needed to make it through that and I would be free. I had five days to live until the end. However, after talking to my cousin during the week she could tell I was not myself. She told me if I didn't tell the psychiatrist everything I was feeling she would be calling 911 and would get them to bring me to the hospital. I went to my appointment on Wednesday and against all odds, told them everything. I was admitted to the psychiatric hospital that day and would remain there for nine weeks.

Being in the hospital allowed me the chance to think, feel and breathe. I was on a cocktail of medications while I was there and I underwent twelve electro-convulsive therapy treatments (yeah, think of the basement of a creepy psych ward and being shocked), lots of one-on-one therapy sessions, many talks with nurses and doctors and a few group therapy sessions. The hospital was my saving grace, my light. Some might think going to the hospital was my rock bottom, but I prefer to look at it as my beginning. I didn't see it at the time but I was so wrong. It was my introduction to finding myself again. Being in the hospital allowed me the chance to start thinking for myself and have enough time alone to take a step back and analyze my life and what was happening in it.

I began to see I was being abused and I started to see that it wasn't all my fault. Maybe I didn't deserve this. Those feelings were some of the hardest I've ever felt. To all of a sudden realize this is not my fault. *But look at the things I've done, the disgusting acts I've performed!* I would think, n*o one can know. I will have no one if they know what I've done.* Still, I remained silent about the abuse. I told no one. No nurses, doctors, friends, or family. I lied ferociously to everyone I knew. I would risk my friendships to protect those secrets. I would risk anything to protect my shame. I couldn't breathe with the grief and shame suffocating me with their debilitating weight, wrapping me in their unforgiving clenched arms never to cease. As long as this weight was on me I was going to remain stuck in the war with my mind. I didn't trust myself to know the truth from lies or right from wrong. I was convinced my mind couldn't be trusted, I was sick, I needed help. I started to open up to my sister-in-law slowly, with much coercion on her part. She visited me often while I was in the hospital and over the weeks I started to become a bit more comfortable with her. I desperately wanted to tell her everything. To beg for her help, to pack my things and have her take me anywhere but my life, yet I couldn't muster the courage to speak. She started to convince me life could be better than this. She had faith in me more than I'd ever had for myself. She saw a strength in me I hadn't seen in years. She believed me. She was and still is one of my most treasured friends—that bond will not break. I came to realize I wasn't sick. I could be trusted, but I did need help. When I started to see the depths of what had happened to me, I immediately wished I had remained in distrust of myself. I wanted my memory to be wrong. I wanted to be "crazy" or "sick." If I were crazy or sick, that would have a cure. A few concoctions of medicine and my mind would be clear and I would be okay again. To my dismay, I could be trusted.

✷ ✷ ✷

Terrified, my stomach clenched so tight it was touching the front of my spine. Nauseous, the fear escalates. The wall felt hard when the back of my head fell against it. Pressed against the wall with nowhere to go, my breath was cut off. The world was closing in on me, darkness overcoming the light as the fight in me was fading and my strength depleting. I held on. Gasping suddenly, my lungs filled with air and my energy rose. I saw my out. I ran toward the door and grabbed my keys on the way out. I dashed across the lawn, hopped over a retaining wall and barrelled into my minivan and peeled out of the driveway. "I'm free. I'm done. I survived. What the fuck did I just do?" I'm not even wearing shoes.

The night I left my marriage was the final straw. Never again would I go back. Not this time. But where do I go from here?

The first few weeks were full of wine and tears. There is no sugar-coating that. I stayed with one of my best friends and her family for those first weeks. I needed the courage to tell my parents. I didn't know what was going to happen. Where would I live? Would I be a waitress forever now? Will my kids be okay? There were so many thoughts racing through my head along with many doubts. I needed my friends to repeatedly tell me I made the right choice. I needed them to say words like rape, abuse, manipulation, gaslighting. I needed to know it was serious. I needed to understand what I had just done. Yet most of all I needed to understand *I was free*. I was safe. I was going to be okay. Above all acceptance of my reality, I needed to feel safe. I needed a home with food in the fridge and a pillow to cry on. I needed a place to feel. I needed to breathe for the first time in seven years. I needed to understand my life was just beginning. I needed to understand this was the first step into a new life. A fresh start. This was my canvas, waiting to be interrupted with vibrant creativity.

I needed to know it was serious. I needed to understand what I had just done. Yet most of all I needed to understand I was free.

I moved in with my parents shortly after I left and had a temporary safe place to lay my head. I had the support and help I needed and could take a few minutes to breathe. The Amber you read about in the beginning isn't the Amber she is now, and the Woman's Crises Service worker watched my story unfold. She has had the pleasure of witnessing me showing emotion and crying for the first time. She got to see me finally *get it*. I finally understood what happened to me. She was there every time I needed her, and every time I needed a kick in the ass. I started to trust again, I started to laugh, and I started to make eye contact. I started to live. I stopped merely staying alive and started to see joy again. I started smiling when my kids smiled and I started hugging them—like really hugging them. I started making deep friendships and making amends where possible for the wrongs I did. I started going to the gym and I quit smoking. I lost sixty pounds. I ran a half marathon. I bought a vehicle. I applied for school and I went. I met an incredible man I now share my life with. I smile. I live now. I don't just survive.

I wish there was a manual I could give to everyone reading this on how I did what I did. How I got out and how I have a life now, but the truth is, it was such a cocktail of people and therapies, restraining orders and family court orders, a house fire, yes a house fire, and everything in between. I went through all of the phases and still go through them. The *"fuck it, where's the wine?"* the *"I've never been more overwhelmed in my life!"* the *"I am an empowered woman, I can do anything!"* I've been through it all. I've sought counselling with a trauma therapist and stay on top of my mental health.

I came to a point in my healing, my acknowledgement and acceptance of what happened where I considered seriously telling the police everything that happened to me. I toyed with the idea for quite some time until I decided to do it. I was doing this for all of the women who thought they couldn't. Standing alongside those who have done it before me and doing it for all the women who will do it after me. Reporting seven years of abuse made me quite possibly the most anxious I'd ever been. I had to tell some friends more details if I was going to do this. I had to tell my mom. If this goes to trial would I even be mentally stable enough to attend? What will this do to the family? What if they don't believe me?

I can honestly say the interview was one of the hardest things I've ever done. I sat in the detective's office in the special victims unit in an uncomfortable chair across from a detective while a video camera poked out of the wall above him. I sat in that room for three hours telling and re-telling my story, clarifying details and answering questions. The next day the detective called and told me there wasn't enough to lay charges, the wording wasn't right, and I gave up again. Thoughts of being crazy and sick came flooding back in, taking up space in my mind they had once occupied. Turns out, it's important to very clearly and loudly use the word "No" if you do not want to do something. It turns out, it's quite difficult in long-term intimate relationships for a charge of that nature to stick. It turned out, or so I thought, I endured all of this to no avail, yet really what I endured all of this for was to share my story to help anyone who needs it.

I've been blessed with an incredible support system that always has my back and is ready to help me back up when I fall. I'm one of the lucky ones. Some have been on "Team Amber" from the start, and some joined along the way. I am dedicated to letting every struggling person know that no matter how dark it gets, there is always *hope*. (I'm aware of how cheesy that sounded). I'm not typically one for cheesy so you've got to trust I mean it when I say it.

There. Is. Always. Hope.

Because of my life experiences, I have learnt an insurmountable amount of lessons and I am learning new lessons all the time. I will never be "complete" because to be complete means to be done growing and if what I've learnt and grown from in the first thirty years of my life is this vast, I could never stop learning and growing. The potential is out there and I'm finally ready to find it. Be tenacious. Be assertive. Be unapologetically you. Say no. Be patient and gracious. Be forgiving.

"Be not afraid, you were born to do this."

- Joan of Arc

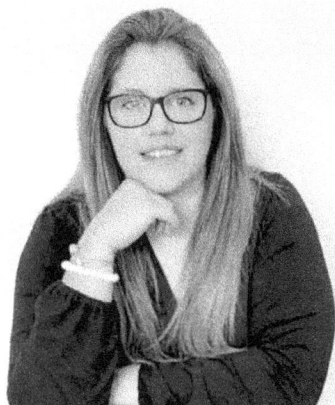

Amber Nicole

Amber Nicole lives in a small town north of Waterloo, Ontario with her three sons and incredible partner Kevin. She has a diploma from Conestoga College in Fitness and Health Promotion and is currently in the midst of Massage Therapy school. Amber is passionate about health and fitness and helping others feel the best they can in their bodies. In her free time, Amber enjoys the outdoors with her family skating, tobogganing, hiking, and camping. On her own, she loves to sit at the piano or hold a guitar and play for hours. Amber is passionate about mental health advocacy and making sure everyone feels heard.

IG: @amber.mlotschek

To Tashia and Adriene, thank you for always being on Team Amber and always letting me feel heard. To Lisa, thank you for being the kick in the ass I needed and for your unending support. To Sarah, thank you for everything you've done for me on my journey so far. I can't wait to see where life takes us. To my parents, thank you for never giving up on me and teaching me that anything is possible. To Kevin and my sons, thank you for giving me a life full of laughter and joy and a reason to get up every day. To everyone else who has been a part of my journey, thank you for everything you have done and taught me along the way and for the role you played in my life.

CHAPTER THIRTEEN

Letting Go

Michelle Hunter

The first time I remember listening to my intuition was also, strangely enough, the last time I would listen to it or even let myself hear it for a very long time. It was April 2016. I was pregnant with my second child and my due date was ten days away. That morning, I hadn't felt him. Not once. I knew. As we drove to the hospital in worried and scared silence, I knew. I knew Cameron was already gone. My second child. My very wanted and longed-for second son, meant to be born in less than two weeks, was already gone.

The most vivid memory. After hearing the doctor tell me that Cameron had passed was hearing my husband cry. Going in to use the bathroom in the hospital room and realizing the gravity of what was happening. I would have to give birth. My milk would come in. The reality that Cameron was gone, there was no changing that, no way to undo that. This harsh reality would continue to bowl me over time after time, day after day, like a punch to the gut. The other facts hadn't even sunk in yet. I would have to plan a funeral for my son and all the firsts

I would never see. How was I supposed to go on after this?

What followed is hard to put into words. A tender silent *hello*. The quietest entrance into the world there would ever be. The silence in the delivery room was deafening. My hopes shattered. I didn't realize it at the time, but until that moment I was holding onto hope that maybe they were wrong. Maybe they could still save him. As I was handed my beautiful boy, born sleeping, perfect as ever, my life was forever divided into before Cameron and after. A few hours to soak in a lifetime of memories we would never get to have. To memorize his face, his perfect hands and feet. Run my finger over his chin dimple, the one matching his big brother's. Handing him back to the nurse hours later, only to walk out of the hospital the following day with a box full of memories, home to a house ready and prepared for a baby. Somehow expected to continue life. Already standing on very shaky ground mentally, the loss of Cameron had me slamming to my bottom.

The months that followed were heavy. That's the only word I can think of to describe it. Getting out of bed each morning was hard. My heart was heavy in my chest, my stomach aching. Everything felt so hard and yet like none of it was real. I think I was very much in a fog of grief and shock. The feeling of loss in my belly felt so empty where Cameron once filled my body. Where so much love once resided but was suddenly missing, my arms were so empty. I didn't know how much empty arms could ache and how grief could physically hurt. It just wasn't fair. I watched the entire world continue and move on around me while my life felt like it was frozen in time. How could I possibly move forward knowing Cameron was never coming home? I couldn't imagine moving on, it didn't seem possible to ever be ok after this. I wanted to scream at everyone I saw. Every "normal" conversation I had to have, anything life required me to attend to. I was screaming inside. Didn't they know? Didn't they know my son died?!

Along with my grief, I carried so much shame. I'm not sure I recognized it as shame at the time. My son died. What must they think? What do they see when they look at me? A failure. They must wonder, "Is it her fault?" I remember going to the doctor to hear the results of the autopsy report, convinced she was going to sit me down and tell me Cameron died because of me. There was no conclusive reason why Cameron was taken from us, but even that didn't release me from the personal hell I was living in. I felt ashamed when I returned to work months later when I should have been on mat leave. I avoided talking to coworkers if I could and kept my head down most of the time. I was the woman who lost her baby. I felt utterly alone. I felt like people were thinking I should have moved on. The thing about shame is that it gets heavy. For me, it fuelled my desire to completely disappear, I didn't want to be seen. Bury my grief, bury my feelings, keep it in. Smother it. Swallow it. Let it eat me up but don't tell anyone how much I am struggling. These emotions were the most intense and heavy I have ever felt. Growing up, my family didn't express emotions freely. We were masters of sweeping things under the rug and hiding emotions, so that's what I did. I kept it all in.

As I mentioned before I wasn't in a great space mentally before Cameron passed away and I had recently reached out for help to a psychologist. I don't want to diminish this to anyone reading. Reaching out for help is huge and it's hard. I suffered in silence for years and years with low self-worth, anxiety and depression. Never speaking my feelings out loud, not to anyone. Not even to my husband. I don't remember what prompted me to make a call to go and see someone, but I don't think it happened by accident. It was only a month or so before we lost Cameron. Having someone to go to during the turmoil of losing a child likely saved my life.

In early October 2016, I became pregnant again and was filled with nothing but fear of losing again. Feeling shame that maybe people thought I was trying to replace Cameron (even though I knew no one ever could). Being unsure if we made the right decision to try again, could I love another baby the way I loved Cameron? Would having another baby mean people would forget about Cameron or think I was all better? Was I supposed to be better?! Would I ever be?!? Then more fear, more guilt, more grief. Imagine waking up every day and feeling like you were encased in cement. That's what I felt. Weighed down. Heavy. Using every ounce of strength I had to move forward and get through the day. Looking back I know I was living in a fog. Caught somewhere between losing Cameron and trying to fast forward to getting Hannah delivered healthy. I couldn't be present in my own life. How could I be when I had so much fear of the future? I was counting down the days I had left in the pregnancy, feeling like I was holding my breath. Once I was far enough along in my pregnancy I started monitoring her movements like crazy. I thought if I just paid enough attention I could prevent another loss. It didn't matter that I was told by doctors there was nothing I could have done or done differently to save Cameron, sometimes these things

The greater my anxiety, the greater my desire to control things.

"just happen." I still felt like I was single-handedly responsible for keeping Hannah alive and getting her here healthy. Each day of pregnancy felt like a year. The thing about anxiety is it makes us believe we need to control everything, that if we can control how things will go everything will be ok. The greater my anxiety, the greater my desire to control things. If I could control enough things, I would feel a false sense of safety.

Let me tell you, trying to control every aspect of my life and especially trying to control things I can't control is exhausting! Physically, mentally and emotionally draining. I believed my own daughter's life was completely in my hands. I had experienced the worst and no one could promise me it wouldn't happen again. I was in a constant state of stress, living on high alert, unable to focus on anything else in my life except the baby in my womb. I couldn't even think about my own needs, the needs of my living son or my husband. It was me and my rainbow baby in the fight for her life and mine. I knew if something happened to her I wouldn't make it either. The anxiety over losing another child was so strong, it occupied my thoughts all day, every day and disrupted every single aspect of my life. In January 2017, my psychologist and OBGYN put me on medical leave from work. It wasn't hard to notice I was not coping well.

Being off work meant I put any shred of attention and energy that wasn't on my pregnancy beforehand (which wasn't much) into keeping Hannah safe. Constantly counting movements, checking the doppler, keep her here. Keep her safe. Being off work and focusing solely on Hannah in my belly was what I thought I needed to do. I could dedicate all my time and energy to her. At the time, I felt like I had a sense of control over the situation as long as I continued to focus on nothing but her.

One particular day I couldn't feel Hannah (or was sure I didn't) and tried the doppler. Nothing but my own heartbeat. Immediately I thought it was happening all over again. I called my husband in and said, "I can't do this again." Already my mind was spinning out, I saw myself having to deliver another stillborn angel and say goodbye all over again. No way would I survive this again. Off to the hospital we go. The nurse's station for check-in was right outside the room where Cameron was delivered silently into this world. Unable to breathe, barely able to get the nurse to understand why I was there. "My son was stillborn last year. I think it's happening again." From that point on, there were many trips to the hospital. If I thought something was wrong and I could just get there in time, I could save her. Prevent, control. Here we are again. As we got closer to the due date, my stress mounted. It felt like at any moment she could be taken from me. I had non-stress tests and extra monitoring but there was so much fear. I didn't enjoy a second of the pregnancy and I wasn't present for very much in my life. My older son was three at the time and I will never get back those moments I missed with him. I was there. My body was there, he physically had a mom, but I know I was not there for him in many ways. I was never present in the moment. There in body but not in mind.

For the last few weeks of my pregnancy, I felt so close yet so far from holding my little girl. I spent days and nights living in the past. I knew that a pregnancy could go from "normal" to over in the blink of an eye. I went to bed one night in April 2016 and felt Cameron wiggling around in my belly and the next morning I never felt him again. When most expectant mothers would be folding baby clothes, getting in those last mornings of sleeping in, and booking newborn photo sessions, I was living frozen in fear I would lose another baby. I knew it could happen, no one could promise me it wouldn't. The safety I felt the moment I heard her heartbeat on the doppler or got an "all good" at a non-stress test lasted just that, a moment. I thought ok she is alive right now, that could change any minute. I was booked for weekly non-stress tests leading to daily towards the end. I was on edge constantly. Not fully present. Not even half present. If I wasn't reliving the passing of Cameron, I was living in fear of losing Hannah. I am ashamed to admit I can't tell you what was going on in the lives of my friends and family or even what my husband and three-year-old son were up to. I knew sometimes babies die and I knew she could too.

Finally, we made it to the day of my C-section. I remember leaving the house, walking into the hospital, lying down on the operating table and still not fully believing I would see my baby girl alive. I felt tears of relief, joy, and renewed grief over what I missed with Cameron the minute I heard her cry. She was here. We did it.

There is a lot of history, too much to analyze in a single chapter of a book but looking back there were a few themes that were prevalent in my childhood, adolescence and early adulthood. Shame, anxiety, and suppression of emotions. I didn't grow up with a lot of confidence or belief in my self-worth. This chapter isn't about why that was or a game of blame but an acknowledgement that was my mindset. I never let myself be seen; hiding was my game. If I hid away, blended into the background no one would see how "not enough" I truly was. I had a poor self-image and an unhealthy body image. I wanted to crawl out of my skin and change everything about myself. Always on a quest to lose weight, be smaller and when I couldn't do that it proved I was worthless. Those feelings of low self-worth spilled into every area of my life. I had a dialogue of negative self-talk running through my head for my entire pre-teen and teen years continuing into adulthood. Growing up we didn't express our emotions. Sadness wasn't shared openly, emotions were buried. Even as an adult, I am still working not to feel shame if I allow someone to see me cry or get emotional. Maybe because I kept everything in, maybe because I felt so much shame, maybe because I didn't believe in myself or value my worth, but I carried a lot of anxiety throughout my life. After experiencing such a traumatic loss of Cameron and the stress of a subsequent pregnancy, I think it's not surprising that I continued to carry anxiety after Hannah was born. I tried to manage my anxiety by controlling everything, trying to see and prevent disasters before they happened, and always preparing for the worst. I never paid attention to myself or my thoughts, my body or my health. I lived to keep order and calm and to prevent more trauma and loss. It is impossible to be present in life while trying to control the future and constantly reliving the past. I would obsessively watch the monitor when Hannah was sleeping, convinced if I didn't, she would die of SIDS. SIDS is a real thing, it happens, so why wouldn't it happen to me? To live in a constant state of fear of losing again and truly believe if I just controlled any variables I could prevent tragedy is *exhausting*. I felt depleted every second of the day but unable to quiet my mind. Always trying to stay two steps ahead, plan, control, prevent. This became a widespread habit in all areas of my life. I was always on high alert, trying to see danger or something unpredictable then play it out in my head, trying to control the outcome. Having things on the to-do list created anxiety until they were done, then something else would be there needing to be tended to. I felt like I had to do everything, complete everything in order to rest. Spoiler alert, the to-do list was never empty therefore the rest never came! I was living on empty all of the time, running on fumes. Never once being aware of what was happening right in front of me and not thinking about what was happening within me. How could I when I was trying to prevent reliving a past trauma by controlling the future?

The feelings of worthlessness I carried through the earlier parts of my life stayed with me too. Perhaps they were even magnified by losing Cameron. I spent a lot of time in my head with a very negative inner dialogue. I cared a lot about what people thought of me (and my inner mean girl told me they didn't think much of me!) I had low self-confidence when it came to my job, my relationships and my body image.

Like many people, I eventually found the wellness world. I started a regime of daily exercise, followed a strict meal plan all under the guise of "health" but really I was trying to chase away the feelings of not being enough and not surprisingly, took comfort in having in having something I could control, manage and predict. I wanted to feel better, look better and ultimately *be* better. I thought if I could follow and stick to a meal plan, exercise every day and lose weight I would be enough. I could finally love myself. I set off on an extremely unhealthy path of controlling everything that went into my mouth, counting calories and tracking everything. I started basing my worth on how well I ate in a day. If I didn't eat according to my meal plan or stick to the 1200 calories I allotted myself, I was just proving that I wasn't enough. I had failed at something else. I kept going, restricting more and controlling more and started losing weight. People noticed and for the first time in my life I felt proud. The compliments I got on my weight loss told me I was doing the right thing; I was getting smaller and now I was on my way to being acceptable to myself and the outside world. I was purely basing my self-worth on the compliments of others, the number on the scale and whether or not I stuck to my meal plan and exercise regime. By the summer of 2017, I was at my lowest weight ever and theoretically, I was on top of the world! I got a high over watching the number on the scale go down. Controlling my weight was my way of chasing acceptance and validation from the outside thinking that is what I needed to do to feel better on the inside. So here I am, at my lowest weight ever, finally achieving what I thought would bring the ultimate self-acceptance and I would finally be worthy! Guess what? Mentally I was lower than ever. I was still consumed with body image thoughts and looking for people to validate my worth. I obsessed about food. The need to control what I was going to eat that day, prep for the next and so on. I needed those compliments so I could tell myself, "I'm ok," "I'm acceptable now." My inner self-critic and negative self-talk were louder than ever! Looking back I know now, I was going about things backwards. I thought if I worked on the outside, the inside would fix itself. Somehow self-love was supposed to come from the scale. What I needed to do was work on the inside, but it took another tragedy for me to finally figure that out.

In 2018 my dad was diagnosed with ALS and slowly became weaker and weaker as the disease took over his body. ALS is 100% fatal and the average survival time from diagnosis is two-five years. The disease was taking everything from him and would continue taking until there was nothing left to take. In December 2020, my dad took a turn for the worse. He was spending more time in bed on his BiPAP machine, losing the ability to use his voice and much of his independence was gone. The thing about ALS is that "as the disease advances and nerve cells are destroyed, your muscles get weaker. This eventually affects chewing, swallowing, speaking and breathing."[2] I was watching this horrific disease kill my father and I was absolutely powerless to stop it. In times of stress or uncertainty, I drop into my old patterns and for me, that was the need to have or try to have control. There was not a thing I could control about the situation with my dad. He was closer to death every day and watching it was excruciating. He requested to spend his last days at home and as a family, we wanted to honour that. I made the difficult decision to take a family medical leave from work to spend my

---

[2] "Understanding ALS."Mayo Clinic. https://www.mayoclinic.org/diseases-conditions/amyo-trophic-lateral-sclerosis/symptoms-causes/syc-20354022)

dad's last days with him. It wasn't an easy decision, but the more I sat with the decision and thought about it, I realized my intuition was loud and clear here. I needed to take this time with my dad. For him, for me, to support my mom as well. This is where I needed to be.

It turned out we had six more months with my dad. Those six months were very difficult for my mom, my siblings and myself. Dad required increasing care and it was difficult to watch him suffer. Knowing there was nothing doctors could do to save my dad, I had to accept I could not control the outcome. This was the first time since losing Cameron (which was different because I didn't see that loss coming) I knew I was about to face a tragic loss and all I could do was watch the speeding train coming. As always I tried to default to control, but this time I started to control my mindset. I can't pinpoint why exactly I made this decision or even if I knew at the time this is what I was doing. Something was telling me I needed to care for myself so I could care for my dad. The process of losing my dad and watching him die was one I had dreaded, even before he was ever sick—typical anxious Michelle here—worrying about losing loved ones was very common for me! Here I was in the middle of one of my greatest fears and my intuition told me I had to do what I could to control how I showed up for my dad and how I cared for my heart and mind during this time. It didn't happen overnight, it was baby steps at first. I was introduced to a mindset practice by a friend, which led me to learn more about various morning practices and breathwork. Each morning after my workout I would allow some time to breathe, focus on nothing but my breath, quiet my mind and take time to breathe in gratitude. This focused time on myself helped me to start letting go of trying to control things outside of me. Finally, I felt control from within. I realized I could control how I showed up every day by bringing calm and stillness to my mornings.

Somehow, something started to change. It wasn't a big change or a drastic change at once, it was small, consistent changes that added up. I think because I wasn't going to work every day and I also wasn't going to my dad's every single day, I had more downtime, quieter moments to realize and notice changes in my mindset. I practiced shifting my mindset by keeping a daily gratitude journal. Studies have shown that practicing gratitude daily increases optimism, relieves stress and over time, people who practice gratitude become more in tune with their surroundings and overall experience more gratitude.[3] Now, I need to be clear here, meditation and gratitude don't equal sunshine and rainbows. Life was still hard. My dad was still dying however, I became more in tune with all aspects of my life and more present. In the past, I had been avoiding and numbing hard feelings and in return was also missing out on a lot of pure joy. Through focusing on myself and incorporating self-care and a morning practice I was present in my life again. Noticing the good in the small moments. One bittersweet thing that sticks out to me on one visit to see my dad is when it was the sweet spot between winter and spring, the snow is almost gone and you can smell spring. It's that beautiful wonderful scent that is hard to describe, that certain feel the breeze has, you just know a new season is around the corner. I immediately felt an immense amount of gratitude and joy for that moment mixed with a deep sadness. At that point, my dad was no longer

3 Miller, Kori D. "14 Health Benefits of Practicing Gratitude According to Science." Positive Psychology. February 4, 2022. https://positivepsychology.com/benefits-of-gratitude/

leaving the house and it shattered me to know he would never feel the spring breeze again. That's the thing about being present. It means we are here for it all, the beautiful and the heartbreaking moments that make up life and all the ordinary moments in between. Brené Brown says, "We cannot selectively numb emotions, when we numb the painful emotions, we also numb the positive emotions." I had avoided and numbed for so long, now I was in it. Feeling it all, experiencing it all. All of those moments are ones I had missed for so long, but here I was, living, present in my own life again, showing up for all these moments we only get to live once. I couldn't go back and make up for lost time, and maybe I didn't want to. It was the struggle that made me who I am today. It was the loss of Cameron that ultimately brought me to the beautiful awareness I was now living. It was my intuition that told me Cameron was gone and now that I had finally welcomed intuition back in, I could live again.

This renewed sense of self and being able to hear my intuition and lean into what I need each day allowed me to heal many aspects of my life. I learned about intuitive eating and was able to, finally, heal from diet culture (again, not overnight and not all at once, it's an ongoing practice), stop hanging on to what other people thought of me and let go of the scale. I started . . . enjoying food and now that I truly knew what I wanted and needed, I started doing more of that! The more I listened to my intuition, the more worthy I felt and guess what? I was enough as I was all along.

Listening to ourselves is a practice, one I am still working on and always will be.

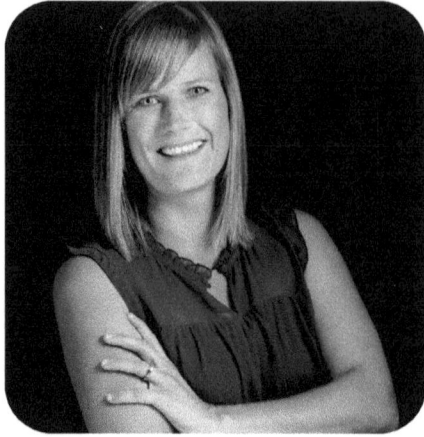

Michelle Hunter

Michelle lives in Kitchener Ontario, Canada with her husband. Together, they have three beautiful children, two living here on earth and one in heaven. She is an elementary school teacher and a certified Mind Body Eating Coach. She is a huge book junkie. She especially binges on thrillers and personal development books. After losing her second-born child, Michelle strives to find moments of gratitude and joy in her day-to-day life.

I want to thank my husband Ian for being my strength when I couldn't find my own. My children for bringing so much joy and love to my life. Also, to all the brave women I have connected with since joining the child loss "club." The inspiration and strength you brought to me during my early days of loss will never be forgotten. To the people in my life that lift me up when I need it most, you know who you are. To Marsha and Sue, for believing in me and helping me find the courage to share my story. I am forever grateful for all the experiences and people that have brought me to the place I am today.

IG @simply_thriving

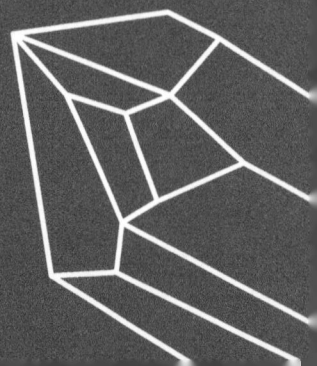

CHAPTER FOURTEEN

The Purge and the Pearl: A Journey Through Bulimia

Jen Lucescu

My first experience with induced purging was when I was two years old. I had eaten a mothball and my mom rushed me to the hospital where I promptly had my stomach pumped. I don't remember this episode, but I imagine my body does. I wonder if I felt relieved as the poison pearl vacated my being. I thought it was a peppermint candy.

At the age of fifteen, this idea of the purge resurfaced. I had struggled with bullying and body shaming throughout elementary school—an all too common pattern that does so much damage in those formative years. As I entered high school, my drive for perfection permeated everything from academics to athletics to personal aesthetics. I had joined the rowing team and found a sense of belonging. As part of a team, we were driven to be strong and powerful women. "Lightweight" women though, meant we had to keep our weight below a certain number during competition season and step on the scale regularly to prove it.2231 The older girls had all of the tips and tricks to help achieve this like taping garbage bags under sweatsuits to go for a run, cabbage soup diets, and the occasional trip to the toilet when we committed the sin of overindulgence.

And hey—if you're going to puke up one cupcake, you might as well eat a whole cake. Thus began my journey with *bulimia nervosa.*

I took a break from rowing after a couple of years to rest my body and make more space for my first boyfriend—a cute boy from the high school in a neighbouring city—and my purging stopped. For a time at least. I started doing yoga with my mom and was introduced to the world of mindfulness. Things were good for a couple of years but jealousy reared its ugly head, destroyed my relationship, and the uncontrollable purging started again. Hidden and shameful, it coloured my whole perspective on life.

It was in full throttle as I entered university then stopped as quickly as it started when I fell in love again in my third year. Sure enough, the binge/purge cycle resurfaced when I moved overseas to South Korea following graduation. My relationship became long-distance, and I was alone again. Living in my own space for the first time in my life, it was easier to hide and indulge my addiction. My daily routine completely revolved around purging: choosing the food, obtaining the food, purging the food and so on. Halfway through my year there, a good friend and I started working out together. I spent weekends away at Buddhist temple stays and meditation courses, and converted to a vegetarian diet. I gathered some useful tools to regain control and bulimia again took a break.

When I returned home to my boyfriend after fifteen months away, no bulimia. Until we broke up and I moved into an apartment above a fish store in the Kensington Market area of Toronto when it began again, this time worse than ever.

I am sure you are seeing the pattern here, of being unable to be alone with or love myself, but I was completely blind to it at the time. Cycling food in and out of my body was a process that gave me bizarre moments of relief but of course, I was spiralling out of control. The cycle of shame and addiction is self-perpetuating and will not resolve on its own. It requires a conscious decision and powerful commitment to alter the behaviour pattern. And a whole bunch of support.

My cycle perpetuated for more than a decade. I knew I had to stop and had managed to do so several times only to find myself right back in it. I planned a trip to India to "get away from it all" and do my Yoga Teacher Training. A few months before leaving, I hit rock bottom. Curled up on the floor of my filthy, cockroach-infested bathroom—I looked in the toilet and saw blood. I felt like I was dying. This path would surely get me there. I wanted to die and upon the surfacing of that thought, an opposite and even more vigorous thought burst through: *I did not want to die*! I was twenty-seven. It was the last time in my life I allowed bulimia but my path to learning how to heal was just beginning. I was spiritually bereft, trying to fill the void, searching for a connection point.

I journeyed to India, the land of the senses, and stayed at an ashram for six weeks to study Yoga and its sister science, Ayurveda. Amongst other things, we were trained in *Panchakarma* cleansing practices such as abdominal oil massage, sweating, nasal and bowel irrigation and, much to my surprise, therapeutic emesis. I experienced relief from these practices such as I had never felt in my life—open channels, vibrant energy and serene bliss. They were done under experienced supervision, only with our informed and willing consent, and together with others

I experienced relief from these practices such as I had never felt in my life—open channels, vibrant energy and serene bliss.

learning the same practices (hello hilarity, as opposed to desolation). These important safeguards set the tone for this new phase of healing in my life, where purging took multiple forms and could be done in ways that are free from shame and safe for my body—including proper preparation and aftercare. I began to understand that my drive to purge was because of densities I felt in my body. Blockages where emotions and memories resided, unseen. And probably a lot of Mac & Cheese.

I learned I was a sensitive person, easily taking on feelings from others near and far. From a very young age, I was tapped into the immensity of the human experience, yet had no tools to name, process or make sense of it. My anxiety often took the form of feeling like the cells of my body could just fly apart at any moment and disappear into the ethers. Food was the only tool I had to ground. I was taking in more than I could digest, literally and figuratively. When you can't take in any more, it has to come out.

When I reflect on my meandering path, I recognize how adversity has been an important guide and teacher. Time and time again, it is in the stagnant feeling of despair I have been willing to let everything go and start anew. To be willing to invite my dark bits into the light so I can take a closer look and create something beautiful out of the available materials.

A therapist of mine once introduced me to the concept of *imaginal cells*, which lie dormant inside our fuzzy caterpillar friends, mere seeds of what is to come. One day they awaken but the caterpillar's immune system doesn't recognize them as "self." There is resistance. A battle ensues. Its life is reduced to goo. And then, in that restful cocoon, the imaginal cells swirl and dream and become. A stunning Monarch emerges, takes some time to understand it has wings, and for the first time takes flight.

It took me decades to understand the parts of myself I share here. It is in the sharing of our stories we find camaraderie, perspective and healing. My purpose in this particular share is to normalize our experiences of shame and empower you to embark on or deepen your healing path. May we find our wholeness as individuals, communities and beyond.

There are tools available to help us move and transform the various energies within us. To peel back the layers of armouring that protect yet restrict us. To liberate us to move towards that within us which is most alive. Let's start at the ground level, a very good place to start indeed.

Are you breathing?
Is that sweet breath reaching every part of you?
Are you moving into those parts?

Even with all of my experiences and acquired wisdom in the realm of breathwork, I still catch myself holding my breath in strange spaces. When I first noticed my breath, I couldn't get it past my diaphragm. In my current work as a Traditional Chinese Medicine (TCM) Practitioner, I see this pattern frequently in my patients.

That sweet nectar of oxygen, that *qi,* that *prana,* that first form of nourishment we take when we are born is meant to be breathed in from each orifice of our body and travel into the deepest core of our womb. We all have a womb space. It is known in Chinese Medicine as the lower *dantian* or "elixir field."

Breathing deep into the belly allows us to ground into the stillest and most stable place within us. It's what we were naturally built to do. When things start feeling out of place, the breath is the first place I remind myself to check. This is accessible medicine we all hold within us. If you're struggling and looking for a first step, consider calling in a teacher to breathe with you. This tool is simple but powerful. Playing with your breathing can cause undesired effects as well. Consider working with a meditation, bodywork, movement expert, or perhaps a therapist.

Learn to breathe.
And then, once you've learned, remember to do it.
Look for the path to open—there is much to be uncovered
in the breath.

I am certain you have heard of or experienced the benefits of meditation. The part that took me a while to understand was there are so many ways to do it. Simply sitting quietly with yourself and breathing for a few minutes every day is transformative, as is lovingly curating living altar spaces in your home or going for an observational walk in the forest. Making a focused intention. Participating in rituals, ceremonies, or drum circles. Committing to a mindful movement practice such as Taiji, Qigong, or Yoga. Kneeling to pray before bed. This is all meditation. All a pathway to relaxing into our own mind/body/spirit connection, a connection that resides more in our steadily beating hearts than in our rapid-firing brains.

I was introduced to Daoist Tea Ceremony nine years ago and have been blessed with many beautiful teachers on that path. Ritualized communion with ethically sourced, wild, old-growth tea leaves has been a way to slow down and tap into my ancient heart to look for guidance and understanding. It has been a way to listen for messages from the Earth herself. I practice inviting younger versions of myself to tea—versions that needed to talk to present-me but had nobody at the time. More recently, I have been sitting with future versions of myself too, as I actively uncover the Crone I move towards, creating Her. Often, I invite those relationships I am struggling with and call in the Ho'Oponopono prayer:

I love you. I'm sorry. Please forgive me. Thank you.

Tears often come when I sit with tea. Tears are a purge. Writing is a purge. Journaling, making lists, penning a story. Like this one. Chasing my monkey mind as I try to settle into meditation is a purge. Anything that gives stagnant energy a pathway out, unblocks the channels and brings us towards clarity and alignment can be considered a purge of unwanted energies.

Our conflicts are a purge too, albeit often disastrous ones if we don't properly recognize them as such. When exploring conflict with another person, it is prudent to set up a safe space, confirm consent to engage with those involved, and utilize breathing and other tools to discharge energy in directions other than at each other. No one likes to get purged on. It's a big mess to clean up.

Shaking is a purge. So is exercise, like jumping on a trampoline with your kids. Dancing is my very favourite, making shapes with my body as I embark on beautiful and sometimes awkward journeys through sound. Sweet movement! Purging out density that obstructs. Moving blood and breath to uncover vibrance. There is a saying many of my teachers recounted throughout my schooling from the ancient Chinese text, the *Huang Di Nei Jing*:

TONG ZE BU TONG; BU TONG ZE TONG.
"If there is free flow there is no pain; if there is pain there is no free flow."

There is so much to discover when we get curious about these bodies. These vessels where our spirit resides. In damaging my body I eventually, thankfully, triggered my self-protection mechanism. I recognized how much my health impacted the way I wanted to show up in the world. My body became a priority, a temple for sacred work, and I became ferocious about protecting it—even more so once I became a mother. Protecting and exploring it.

An eclectic range of tools and opportunities are available to us life-livers. The worldwide *Ecstatic Dance* community is a sober and supportive haven for exploring movement and connection. *Axis Syllabus* workshops are unique and informative investigations into the structure and potential of the human form. *Radical Aliveness* workshops are a kind of group therapy session in which the goal is to unlock our spontaneity and authenticity. *Somatic Processing* works directly on the nervous system by learning to flow between states of relaxation and discharge. *Qigong, Kung Fu and Yoga* develop mastery in relaxing into our alignment and properly guiding energy through. These are but a few—there is so much more! Choose your adventure.

In all cases, I strongly recommend looking for guides that honour the importance of the "container." This refers to the defined space and time allotted for the work so we can enter in consciously and have clear closure. Safe space-holders for individual or group therapeutic encounters commit to open communication, informed consent, confidentiality, clear boundaries and a channel for post-experience integration.

This is important as the work of purging can be gruelling and relentless. With these tools, we often unearth something we feel unprepared to manage on our own. There are parts of the human experience that feel unbearable and it is all too easy to be immobilized by the feeling we are responsible for "fixing" things. Sometimes, all we can do is witness. Name what we see and notice how we feel and then consider how we can best move forward as kind, connected people. We need these tools to go inward and we also need to be able to come back and be present to what is in front of us. When we understand the temporary nature of a situation, we can allow ourselves to let go and go deeper in our practice. Strong containers also help connect us to the wisdom that *every situation is temporary.*

Trust increases as experience is gained on the path, so long as our experiences feel safe. With masterful guidance, our most challenging encounters show us our courage. We can discover our resilience and thus begin to de-armour ourselves and approach our vulnerable core. Tension dissolves and we learn to connect to source power. The spiritual path is one of direct revelation unique to each individual. It must be a lived experience to bear fruit.

This is how I learn to follow my heart: I ask a question, listen for the slightest message, take decisive action to follow that instinct, then reflect on it later. Through this process, the messages become more clear and I find myself less frequently stuck in the stagnant waters of indecision.

Once, in a Radical Aliveness workshop I attended, we were practicing listening to the movements our bodies were craving. I named a desire to be wildly spun around a stable point. That was the movement, the purge, that my body *wanted*. Members of the group tried clasping my hand and flinging me around but the walls of the room felt too small, the strength of my tether too tame. I was frustrated. Unsatisfied. I let go. I began spinning like a whirling dervish while the rest of the group hustled to form a ring around the room boundaries to keep a safe space. I spun and spun until I collapsed in a blissful heap on the floor. I had satisfied the answer my body was searching for. I needed trust to let go into my wildness, to discover the tether I was seeking could only be found within myself.

We can practice completing our stories.
We can find resolution by feeling our emotions all the way through.

Sometimes I want to curl up into a ball and sob—to hold my grief and hide it under warm covers. But this solidifies my outer boundary and so buries it deeper within my body; my body that is now shaking with stifled sound so as not to alarm my loved ones. So instead I sprawl backwards over a bolster, opening my arms to the heavens, and let out the ugly wails. The growls and screams of frustration. The unrecognizable sounds of feelings I can't even identify. It is not the time to analyze what is happening but simply to give myself permission. The more voice I give my emotions, the more sound comes through. Sound has a wisdom of its own when mental constructs fail. I exhaust myself, searching for any more tension in my body that wants to make noise. There is nothing. Nothing but the tingling warmth of bliss.

Movement and somatic therapy have brought me the massive learning in that *I don't need to hold things in my physical body* and introduced me to methods of finding these things and moving them out. I received invitations to expand into the container that is my soul, which can hold so much more. From dense to sublime. This is the work of alchemy and transformation.

The work is never done. It takes a lifetime. Lifetimes, maybe. Practice is building a new pattern into memory, instead of repeating destructive patterns. We learn new tools and practice them and *let it be hard* so when things get hard again we have new reference points to when we struggled and were supported and saw it through. "Doing the work" doesn't mean you are not going to struggle anymore. It might actually feel like you are struggling *more* because now you have more awareness. Instead of bypassing and distracting, you are now noticing how much tension lives in your body. You are uncovering the deep, seedy underbelly of shadow. We offer ourselves, our embodied lives, to process it in mindful ways so it is less likely to surface in more insidious unconscious ways.

I want to acknowledge here we must deal with the psychological undertone of our issues. Psychotherapy is a hugely important and irreplaceable tool I believe everyone can benefit from, though it can take time and commitment to find the right therapist. It needs to be someone who feels safe and connected and delivers their observations in a way that resonates with you and empowers you to be hopeful about your choices.

Be specific. I have sought different therapists depending on the experience I was trying to integrate at the time: Relational separations, lack of career purpose, ecological distress, or a struggling child. Most therapists are willing to have a free introductory conversation so you can see if it's a good fit for both of you and enter the relationship with respect and consent. Look for trauma-informed care, which understands the interrelation between trauma and symptoms of trauma such as mental distress, disordered eating, addictions and other self-harming behaviours.

Trauma is about the loss of connection to ourselves, our bodies, our communities and also to the natural world around us and beyond. It can happen incrementally and be hard to recognize. It can be passed down through generations. In my journey, it has been difficult but rewarding to put myself in the vulnerable space of being truly seen, to uncover the patterns that do not serve me and to have guidance in choosing another way, for myself and all my relations. Therapy is essential self-care and, in a just society, should be accessible to everyone as a means of breaking abusive cycles.

I had a partner for more than a decade that struggled with substance abuse, and through that process, I became intimate with the AA (Alcoholics Anonymous) and NA (Narcotics Anonymous) 12 step programs. Common themes in that process include honesty, humility, surrender, prayer, meditation, internal reflection, relationship reparations and connection. It is so hard, this inner work. It requires we approach what we are trying to cover up and expose the most vulnerable parts of ourselves. Modern society puts value on the appearance of strength and charisma. The undesirable bits are left to find their way in the shadows.

Trauma happens to all of us. It is the nature of being human. We suffer in these mortal human lives and are confronted with ideas that are too big for us to cope with. The question is not, "How do we avoid it?" But instead "What do we do when we encounter it?"

I didn't speak a word of my struggle with bulimia to anyone at the time

I was going through it. Perhaps there were tools and supports available but I didn't access them. The internet had just become a thing, so I crept online chat rooms looking for support, and essentially found more tips and tricks for hiding. I put my fingers down my throat and silenced myself. I spent more than a decade in a perpetual state of dehydration. I burned my esophageal tract with stomach acids and degraded my teeth which require special care and strengthening to this day.

Only now can I see the correlation between my throat energy centre and weak boundaries. The healing power of my voice—sharing, singing, sounding, saying no, saying *yes*—has helped repair the damage done. I changed my life by changing the way I speak to myself. I continue to change my life by considering the way I speak to myself and listening for my authentic truth.

Our rest is sacred. We purge to clear space and then relax into that void to imagine, to dream what we want to be. Evolution requires us to get ourselves out of the productivity and self-improvement trap and swim in the waters of our creativity. We have big feelings to feel, big challenges to overcome. Our distress is showing us our love. It is saying we have too many things on the to-do list, yet we're neglecting the most important necessities of life. Love is calling on us to be more careful with this precious life we have been given.

The pattern of bulimia nervosa, and many other addictions, is supremely wasteful. Wasteful of time, money, food, health, vibrance, energy. I had to feel that compulsive consumption so I could loathe it. So I could understand I was healthier when I utilized awareness and discernment. Generally speaking, evaluating consumption is a requirement for allowing our ailing planet to regenerate.

In my recovery, I continue to dance on the line between easeful intuition and neurotic tendencies. The ethics of food can uncover devastating realities. There is enough trauma in there to spark a wide range of eating disorders.

How are the animals treated which provide sustenance for us humans?
What chemicals and toxins are hiding in our foods?
Are we devastating or supporting communities by importing exotic goods?

How can we move through the understanding that nourishing ourselves may be harming another life?

I have spiralled in many of these spaces and grappled for control through restriction, only to feel like nothing is safe to eat. I found relief connecting to local farmers and food sources and nutrition models that are grounded in moderation, enjoyment and personalization based on individual constitution and connection to the natural world with its changing seasons.

Our bodies and nature are not separate.
The situation is always changing.
Our choices matter.

We are actively creating the world we are living in through each thought and action. I now live in an intentional farming community and understand the immense amount of work required to plant, grow, harvest and preserve food. Our food workers are grossly underpaid and overworked. There is medicine in learning to treasure every morsel and give back to the soil in gratitude. Proper nourishment boosts the element of Earth in our bodies and gives us stability.

> *"The food you eat can be either the safest and most powerful form of medicine or the slowest form of poison."*
>
> -Ann Wigmore

And so it goes for everything we take in, through all of our orifices— is it medicine or poison? Alcohol was one of the very first medicines. Tobacco is a sacred plant. Movies and TV series can be great art. But are we considering the purpose *each time* we consume? Can we feel the movements within our bodies? Are we using it to connect? Or disconnect? Our habits are so frequently a slow and insidious form of self-harm. Perhaps the greatest commitment we can make to ourselves is to find stability and alignment, in body and in action.

I have found hope and courage in gathering various tools so there are different angles to approach a block or a challenge. Whatever methods we use, it's essential to continually assess whether it's working for us. Any information we receive needs to go through the filter of our heart-mind as we learn to self-lead and show discernment. Take what works and leave what doesn't, be ready to pivot.

Our bodies are made of energy, pulsing to the interplay of breath and movement. What is your way in? All senses move the energy.

Sound—listen, sing, chant, drum, bang a gong, shake a rattle, play guitar, join a sound bath. *Move the energy.*

Smell—burn incense, discover flower essences, breathe with a tree, simmer a nutritious soup. *Move the energy.*

Taste—experience pure water, invigorating spice, subtle tea, personalized herbs. *Move the energy.*

Sight—walk in the woods, observe an animal, candle gaze, paint your visions. *Move the energy.*

Touch—lay skin to the soil, treat yourself to bodywork, have a long hug, go skinny dipping. *Move the energy.*

And, Beyond—meditate, visualize, journey, pray, love. Follow the stars. *Move the energy.*

Choose any door and make a heartfelt request for the right guide to appear. Give deep gratitude for the messages you find along the way. Forgive yourself when you feel lost. Forgive others for their sometimes misguided directions. Learn to lead yourself on your path and ask for help when you need it. Rest. Reflect. Repeat.

These practices make me a healer. Not because I have any magical powers or professed mastery but because *I am* a human that *is* healing.

In my commitment to that process, each moment is abundant in meaning and feeling. I learn from all beings, all the time. When I share a healing space, food, health, vibrance, and energy with someone, we are both engaged in that process.

I see you. I understand your struggle. You are not alone. This is how we relax into it.

I want to invite you into the courageous warrior work of getting to know yourself. Of witnessing how messy and flawed and glorious we all are. Of following the primitive impulse towards the choice to be alive. When I sit with previous versions of myself, I can see many places where there was a scared and isolated girl who thought it would be so much easier to just not exist anymore. And in those spaces there often came a clue, a guide, a curious message inviting me into the mystery. This is my invitation to you.

In diving deeper into my body, I forge a relationship with the pearl within my womb which Sages through time describe with reverence. It is an inner compass and creative energy source that can be touched upon by my will and it is up to me to keep it alive. My ongoing internal commitment. This pearl is not the poison mothball of my infancy—it is the medicine of living a meaningful life.

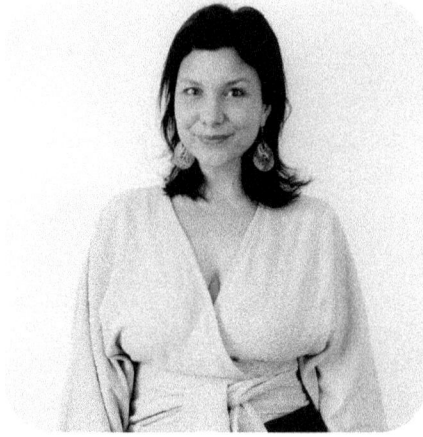

Jen Lucescu

Jen Lucescu is a hedgewitch and shapeshifter that has studied meditation, movement and medicine for more than twenty years. A devoted student of the rose, the leaf and the drum, she courageously hones her skills through practice, trial and error. She is deeply blessed to mother a feisty daughter and be mothered by a spiritually-guided Crone, as they walk the path of ancestral healing together. As a Traditional Chinese Medicine Practitioner with a committed Qigong practice, she moves through life with the ebb and flow of the seasons. She currently lives embedded in nature in an intentional farming ecovillage community in Southwestern Ontario with her beloved daughter, partner, cat and bees. Jen would like to acknowledge that the land on which she writes, gardens, lives and loves is the traditional territory of the Mississaugas of the Credit First Nation. She is grateful to have the honour of stewarding these lands and by doing so, shows her respect to its first inhabitants. She supports the continued conversation between all peoples to find truth, reconciliation, and justice now and in the future. This is Jen's first published work. Although, if the fork in the head-line of her palm is any indication, there will be more to come.

IG @oohletmesee

I would like to acknowledge my teachers, protectors and guides, in all of their brilliant forms, throughout all of my life. May all beings, everywhere, be happy and be free.

Final Words

Thank you for taking the time to read this collection of real-life body stories from these courageous authors. They have shared their experiences, emotions, life traumas, loss, challenges, and triumphs. No longer hiding behind or stuck in their stories, their fears or the judgements of others. They share their stories to pass on their lessons, solutions and perspectives to guide you with your journey or challenges. It is the simple yet profound act of "paying it forward" that they embody fully. Their stories are here on the earth to support others. This is the ripple effect we choose to be a part of, and you can too.

If you feel called to share a body story and know deep down you are meant to be a published author in one of our next collaborative books, please feel free to reach out to Marsha and Sue and continue to honour these brave humans who shared their stories with you by sharing them with others. Pass this book on to a close friend, share a quote or lesson you gathered (should that feel safe to do) on your social accounts, or start a book reading with a group of friends.

Because, *Every Body*. . .Holds a Story.

Additional Resources

This section provides additional resources with books, links, journal prompts, and other helpful information that contributed to each author's journey. Take what you need and enjoy!

Books

- *Ask and It Is Given* by Esther and Jerry Hicks
- *Atomic Habits* by James Clear
- *Beautifully Brave* by Sarah Pendrick
- *Body Kindness* by Rebecca Scritchfield
- *Breaking the Habit Of Being Yourself, How to Lose your Mind and Create a New One* by Dr. Joe Dispenza
- *By The Moon A Quote Book By Spirit Daughter* by Jill Wintersteen
- *Clarity & COnnection* by Yung Pueblo
- *Daring Greatly* by Brené Brown
- *Happy Days* by Gabby Bernstein
- *Healing With Whole Foods: Asian Traditions and Modern Nutrition.* 3rd ed., rev., updated, and expanded. Berkeley, Calif.: North Atlantic Books, 2002. Print.
- *Health at Every Size* by Linda Bacon
- *Heart Talk* by Cleo Wade
- *Intuitive Eating* Evelyn Tribole M.S. R.D, Elyse Resch M.S. R.D. F.A.D.A.
- *Inward* by Yung Pueblo
- *Just Breathe by Mastering Breathwork* by Dan Brulé
- *Journey To The Heart* by Melody Beattie
- *Mindset* by Carol S. Dweck, Ph. D
- *The Four Agreements* by Don Miguel Ruiz
- *The Gifts of Imperfection* by Brené Brown
- *The Great Canadian Woman Series* of books

- *The Power of Intention* by Dr. Wayne Dyer
- *The Untethered Soul* by Michael Singer
- *The Untethered Soul Guided Journal* by Michael Singer
- *The Intelligent Patient Guide to Breast Cancer.* Intelligent Patient Guide Ltd., Gelmon, K., Kuusk, U., McCready, D., & Olivotta, I. (2012).

Links

Alternative Treatments:

breastcancerconqueror.com/

Cone biopsy

cancer.ca/en/treatments/tests-and-procedures/cone-biopsy

Dissociative Amnesia

integrativelifecenter.com/wellness-blog/childhood-trauma-memory-loss/

Doppler

A fetal Doppler is a test that uses sound waves to check your baby's heartbeat.

www.webmd.com/baby/fetal-doppler#1

Dr. Annette Richard's website for breast cancer patients:

https://www.faceitbreastcancer.com/dr-annette-richard

Eatwell Centre—private centre in Ontario

Online treatment across Canada, anyone can call for resources, https://www.
eatwellhealthcentre.ca/

Emotional Freedom Technique (EFT)

Also known as tapping is an alternative therapy for anxiety, post-traumatic
stress disorder and many other conditions. Tapping draws on the ancient
Chinese practice of acupuncture which teaches that the body's energy travels
along specific pathways.

www.medicalnewstoday.com and www.webmd.com

EMDR Childhood Trauma and Re-Processing through EMDR

https://cancer.ca/en/treatments/tests-and-procedures/cone-biopsy

Endometriosis

https://integrativelifecenter.com/childhood-trauma-memory-loss/

https://www.hopkinsmedicine.org/health/conditions-and-diseases/
endometriosis

Father/Daughter Relationship Articles

www.psychologytoday.com/us/blog/
behavior-problems-behavior-solutions/202012/what-girl-needs-her-dad

NEDIC—National Eating Disorder Info Centre

https://nedic.ca/

Live Blood Analysis

A simple procedure for obtaining a quick assessment of your blood. A drop of your blood is analyzed under a microscope and can identify vitamin and mineral deficiencies, toxicity, and tendencies toward allergic reaction, excess fat circulation, liver weakness and hydration status.

My girls cream

mygirlscream.com/brands/My-Girls%E2%84%A2-Skin-Care.html

Ozone

https://www.youtube.com/c/DrOSolutions

Non-stress test

A non-stress test is a common prenatal test used to check on a baby's health. During a non-stress test, the baby's heart rate is monitored to see how it responds to the baby's movements. The term "non-stress" refers to the fact that nothing is done to place stress on the baby during the test. Typically, a non-stress test is recommended when it's believed that the baby is at an increased risk of death. A non-stress test may be done after 26 to 28 weeks of pregnancy. https://www.mayoclinic.org/tests-procedures/nonstress-test/about/pac-20384577

Rainbow baby

A rainbow baby is a name coined for a healthy baby born after losing a baby due to miscarriage, infant loss, stillbirth, or neonatal death. www.healthline.com/health/pregnancy/rainbow-baby

Reiki

A form of energy healing therapy.

Tribal Trade Company

www.facebook.com/TribalTradeCo/

Verbal/Emotional Abuse

http://www.ashleighspatienceproject.com/abuse-types-and-cycle-wheel.html

Visanne

www.medbroadcast.com/drug/getdrug/visanne

Podcasts and videos

Ancestral Healing Podcast

mythicmedicine.love/podcast/

Hydration and Water Blessings

www.waterislife.love/

My Qigong Teacher (Permission given)

www.claireturnerreid.com/

My Reiki Teacher (Permission given)

www.donnawilding.com/

Traditional Chinese Medicine School

www.octcm.com/

Radical Aliveness

radicalaliveness.org/

Ecstatic Dance

ecstaticdance.org/

Apps

AUDIBLE books

Great when you're on the move/commute/working out.

INSIGHT TIMER

Lots of free meditations and yoga.

Global Grounding Community

Myofascial Release, community, support.

OTHERSHIP

Breathwork App.

Journal prompts:

How do I want to feel today?

What can I do to ensure I feel that today?

Where do I need support today?

How can I support myself today?

My intention(s) for today is/are . . .

_____

_____

_____

_____

What is one thing I can do, right now, to live from a higher vibration?

_____

_____

_____

_____

How am I feeling today?

_____

_____

_____

_____

List 3-5 things you are grateful for or appreciate—great way to start and finish your day.

_____

_____

_____

_____

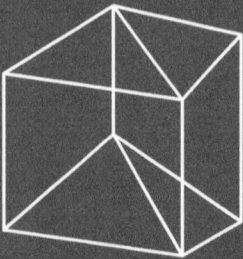

Glossary

We created this glossary of terms for quick access to reference when needed.

All definitions provided in this glossary are from the Merriam-Webster Medical Dictionary (https://www.merriam-webster.com/medical). Any additional definitions have their website sourcing for further information.

Adenomyosis endometriosis

Especially when the endometrial tissue invades the myometrium

Additional definition: is a condition in which the lining of the uterus (the endometrium) breaks through the muscle wall of the uterus. www.*webmd.com*

Amyotrophic Lateral Sclerosis (ALS)

A rare progressive degenerative fatal disease affecting the motor neurons, usually beginning in middle age, and characterized especially by increasing and spreading muscular weakness and atrophy—abbreviation ALS—called also Lou Gehrig's disease

Ayahuasca

A psychoactive beverage containing dimethyltryptamine that is prepared especially from the bark of a woody vine (*Banisteriopsis caapi* of the family Malpighiaceae) and the leaves of a shrubby plant (*Psychotria viridis* of the family Rubiaceae) of South America.

NOTE: Ayahuasca produces hallucinations and euphoria and is used chiefly for religious, ritualistic, and medicinal purposes. Alkaloids present in ayahuasca inhibit the breakdown of dimethyltryptamine in the liver and gastrointestinal tract by monoamine oxidase.

Additional definition: is a psychoactive tea that originates from the Amazon region. Psychoactive substances affect the brain and cause people to experience changes in their mood, thinking, and behaviour. Traditional healers in several South American countries use the tea for its reported healing properties.

This tea is a brew made from the stalks of the Banisteriopsis caapi vine and Psychotria viridis shrubs. *www.healthline.com and*

https://en.m.wikipedia.org

Ayurveda

A form of alternative medicine that is the traditional system of medicine of India and seeks to treat and integrate body, mind, and spirit using a comprehensive holistic approach especially by emphasizing diet, herbal remedies, exercise, meditation, breathing, and physical therapy.

Bilevel positive airway pressure

A technique that is used for relieving breathing problems (such as those associated with sleep apnea or congestive heart failure) by pumping a flow of air through the nose to prevent the narrowing or collapse of air passages or to help the lungs expand and that differs from continuous positive airway pressure by pumping air at a reduced pressure during each exhalation. One alternative is a unit that provides what is known as *bilevel positive airway pressure*, or BIPAP. It delivers more pressure when you inhale and less when you exhale, and tends to be better tolerated than CPAP.

—Joseph Kaplan

—abbreviation *BiPAP, BIPAP, BiPap, BPAP, BPap*

Body Psychotherapy

An approach to psychotherapy which applies basic principles of somatic psychology (focusing on therapeutic and holistic approaches to the body) used to engage the relationship between mind, body, brain, and emotions.

https://integrativepsych.co/ and https://en.mikipedia.org

Bulimia Nervosa

A serious eating disorder characterized by compulsive overeating usually followed by self-induced vomiting or laxative or diuretic abuse, and is often accompanied by guilt and depression.

Chakra

Any of several points of physical or spiritual energy in the human body according to yoga philosophy.

Additional definition: refer to various energy centres in your body that correspond to specific nerve bundles and internal organs. The seven major chakras run from the base of your spine to the top of your head. If these energy centres get blocked, you may experience physical or emotional symptoms related to a particular chakra.

www.healthline.com

Cone Biopsy Dysfunction (Conization)

The electrosurgical excision of a cone of tissue from a diseased uterine cervix.

Cortisone: a glucocorticoid $C_{21}H_{28}O_5$ of the adrenal cortex used in synthetic form especially as an anti-inflammatory agent.

Additional definition: is a steroid drug. It helps decrease swelling and inflammation in your body. It works by stopping the release of molecules that cause inflammation. This also stops your body from having an immune response. *www.healthline.com*

Caution: Local corticosteroid injection has complications such as infection,

sepsis, facial flushing, hypopigmentation, perilymphatic atrophy, bleeding, tendon

rupture, steroid flare, soft tissue atrophy, and hypersensitivity reaction. In this

case study, the patient had hypopigmentation, subcutaneous fat and muscle

atrophy, and nerve injury.

https://www.ncbi.nlm.nih.gov/pmc/articles/PMC3903862/

Dissociative amnesia

One of a group of conditions called dissociative disorders. Dissociative
disorders are mental illnesses that involve disruptions or breakdowns of
memory, consciousness, awareness, identity, and/or perception. When one or
more of these functions is disrupted, symptoms can result. These symptoms
can interfere with a person's general functioning, including social and work
activities, and relationships.

EFT (Emotional Freedom Technique)

Also known as tapping is an alternative therapy for anxiety, post-traumatic
stress disorder and many other conditions. Tapping draws on the ancient
Chinese practice of acupuncture which teaches that the body's energy travels
along specific pathways.

www.medicalnewstoday.com and www.webmd.com

Energy Work or Energy Healing

It is based on the belief that the body is permeated by an energy field that can affect our health and well-being. Types of energy healing includes several modalities including but not limited to Reiki, acupuncture, touch therapy, EFT tapping, somatic body work, chakra balancing, crystal healing, shamanic healing, breathwork and so much more. www.*healthline.com*

Endometriosis

The presence and growth of functioning endometrial tissue (the mucous membrane lining the uterus) in places other than the uterus that often results in severe pain and infertility.

Eye Movement Desensitization and Reprocessing (EMDR) therapy

An extensively researched, effective psychotherapy method proven to help people recover from trauma and other distressing life experiences, including PTSD, anxiety, depression, and panic disorders. https://www.emdria.org/about-emdr-therapy/

Fascia

Fascia is a layer of connective tissue that surrounds every muscle, bone, blood vessel, nerve, and organ in the body. It is connected, head-to-toe, without interruption.

Fibromyalgia

A chronic disorder characterised by widespread pain, tenderness, and stiffness of muscles and associated connective tissue structures that is typically accompanied by fatigue, headache, and sleep disturbances.

Additional information: Researchers believe that fibromyalgia amplifies painful sensations by affecting the way your brain and spinal cord process painful and non-painful signals. *www.mayoclinic.org*

Glaucoma

A disease of the eye marked by increased pressure within the eyeball that can result in damage to the optic disk and gradual loss of vision.

Additional definition: is a condition that damages your eye's optic nerve. It gets worse over time and is linked to a buildup or pressure inside your eye. Glaucoma tends to run in families and usually does not surface until later in life. *www.webmd.com*

Homeostasis

A relatively stable state of equilibrium or a tendency toward such a state between the different but interdependent elements or groups of elements of an organism, population, or group.

Hysterectomy

A surgical removal of the uterus with or without other organs or tissues. In a total hysterectomy, the uterus and cervix is removed.

Lissencephaly (smooth brain)

The condition of having a smooth appearance on the surface of the brain. *Specifically* : an abnormality of brain development marked by the presence of a smooth cerebral cortex with few or no convolutions.

Molar Pregnancy (hydatidiform mole)

A mass in the uterus that consists of enlarged edematous degenerated chorionic villi growing in clusters resembling grapes, that typically develops following fertilisation of an enucleate egg, and that may or may not contain fetal tissue.

Nervous System

The bodily system that in vertebrates is made up of the brain and spinal cord, nerves, ganglia, and parts of the receptor organs and that receives and interprets stimuli and transmits impulses to the effector organs.

Sympathetic

the part of the autonomic nervous system that contains chiefly adrenergic fibres and tends to depress secretion, decrease the tone and contractility of smooth muscle, and increase heart rate.

Parasympathetic

The part of the autonomic nervous system that contains chiefly cholinergic fibres, that tends to induce secretion, to increase the tone and contractility of smooth muscle, and to slow heart rate, and that consists of a cranial and a sacral part.

Additional definition: parasympathetic nervous system is responsible for the body's rest and digestion response when the body is relaxed, resting, or feeding. It basically undoes the work of sympathetic division after a stressful situation. The main purpose is to conserve energy to be used later and to regulate bodily functions like digestion, salivation, tears, and urination. *www. sciencedirect.com and https://en.m.wikipedia.org*

Ophthalmology

A branch of medical science dealing with the structure, functions, and diseases of the eye.

Ophthalmologists

They are medical doctors who specialise in the diagnosis and treatment of eye and vision problems. www.*webmd.com*

Ozone therapy

Ozone therapy refers to the process of administering ozone gas into your body to treat a disease or wound. Ozone is a colourless gas made up of three atoms of oxygen ($O3$).

More information can be found at www.healthline.com/health/ozone-therapy and www.youtube.com/c/DrOSolutions

Past life regression

It is a method that uses hypnosis to recover what practitioners believe are memories of past lives or incarnations. https://en.m.*wikipedia.org*

Postpartum Depression

Involving intense psychological depression that typically occurs within one month after giving birth, lasts more than two weeks, and is accompanied by other symptoms (such as social withdrawal, difficulty in bonding with the baby, and feelings of worthlessness or guilt).

"Strictly defined, *postpartum depression* is diagnosed by the criteria for major depression—overwhelming feelings of sadness, guilt or worthlessness for at least two weeks—beginning sometime in the month after the baby is born."
—Jill U. Adams

". . . 10 to 20 percent of new mothers in the United States feel so depressed within six months of childbirth that they have trouble with normal functioning. This is *postpartum depression* . . . and it can occur after the birth of any child."—Andrew Weil

". . . it turns out that men can also have *postpartum depression*, and its effects can be every bit as disruptive—not just on the father but on mother and child."—Richard A. Friedman

Piriformis

A muscle that arises from the front of the sacrum, passes out of the pelvis through the greater sciatic foramen, is inserted into the upper border of the greater trochanter of the femur, and rotates the thigh laterally.

Additional definition: this muscle is a flat, band-like muscle located in the buttocks near the top of the hip joint. This muscle is important in lower body movement as it stabilises the hip joint and lifts and rotates the thigh away from the body. www.*wedmd.com*

Psoas Major

The larger of the two psoas muscles that arises from the anterolateral surfaces of the lumbar vertebrae, passes beneath the inguinal ligament to insert with the iliacus into the lesser trochanter of the femur, and serves especially to flex the thigh.

Psoas Minor

The smaller of the two psoas muscles that arises from the last dorsal and first lumbar vertebrae and inserts into the brim of the pelvis, that functions to flex the trunk and the lumbar spinal column, and that is often absent.

Additional definition: a tight psoas muscle can cause a multitude of problems such as chronic back pain, poor posture, bloating, constipation, functional leg length discrepancy, leg rotation, sciatica, an obtunded abdomen, and can affect the drainage of lymph. The psoas muscle can be the answer to not only your back pain but also our digestive issues. *opmed.doximity.com and www. my.clevelandclinic.org*

Psilocybin

A hallucinogenic indole $C_{12}H_{17}N_2O_4P$ obtained from a fungus (such as *Psilocybe mexicana* or *P. cubensis* synonym *Stropharia cubensis*).

"Studies using *psilocybin* are also showing great promise relieving the symptoms of depression, PTSD, eating disorders and drug misuse disorders."

— David E. Carpenter, *Forbes*, 18 Jan. 2022

Reiki

A system of touching with the hands based on the belief that such touching by an experienced practitioner produces beneficial effects by strengthening and normalising certain vital energy fields held to exist within the body.

Stillbirth

The birth of a deceased fetus.

Additional definition: stillbirth is the delivery, after the 20th week of pregnancy, of a baby who has died. Loss of a baby before the 20th week of pregnancy is called a miscarriage. A baby is stillborn in about 1 in 200 pregnancies. www.webmd.com/baby/understanding-stillbirth-basics

Sudden Infant Death Syndrome (SIDS)

A death of an apparently healthy infant usually before one year of age that is of unknown cause and occurs especially during sleep —abbreviation *SIDS*

Additional definition: the unexplained death, usually during sleep, of a seemingly healthy baby less than a year old. SIDS is sometimes known as crib death because the infants often die in their cribs.

www.mayoclinic.org/diseases-conditions/sudden-infant-death-syndrome/symptoms-causes/syc-20352800

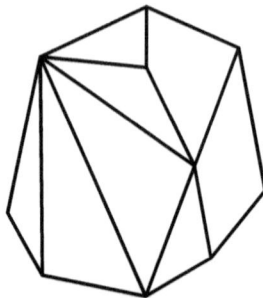

Thyroid

A large bilobed endocrine gland of vertebrates lying at the anterior base of the neck and producing especially the hormones thyroxine and triiodothyronine. Additional definition: a butterfly-shaped gland that sits low on the front of the neck. The thyroid secretes several hormones, collectively called thyroid hormones. The hormones act throughout the body, influencing metabolism, growth as well as development, and body temperature. *www.webmd.com*

Tonsillectomy

The surgical removal of the tonsils. Tonsils are either of a pair of prominent masses of lymphoid tissue that lie one on each side of the throat between two folds of soft tissue that bound the fauces.

Uvula

The pendent fleshy lobe in the middle of the posterior border of the soft palate. Additional definition: It secretes large amounts of saliva that keep your throat moist and lubricated. It also helps keep food or fluids from entering up in the space behind your nose when you swallow. Your uvula is also considered an organ of speech. *www.webmd.com*

Vagus nerve

Either of the 10th pair of cranial nerves that arise from the medulla oblongata and supply chiefly the viscera especially with autonomic sensory and motor fibres. borrowed from New Latin *vagus nervus*, literally, "wandering nerve,"; so called from its multiplicity of connecting points in the neck, thorax, and abdomen.

Vertigo

A sensation of motion in which the individual or the individual's surroundings seem to whirl dizzily.

Whole Genome Sequencing

It is a comprehensive method for analysing entire genomes. Genomic information has been instrumental in identifying inherited disorders, characterising the mutations that drive cancer progression, and tracking disease outbreaks. Rapidly dropping sequencing costs and the ability to produce large volumes of data with today's sequencers make whole-genome sequencing a powerful tool for genomics research. https://www.illumina.com/techniques/sequencing/dna-sequencing/whole-genome-sequencing.html

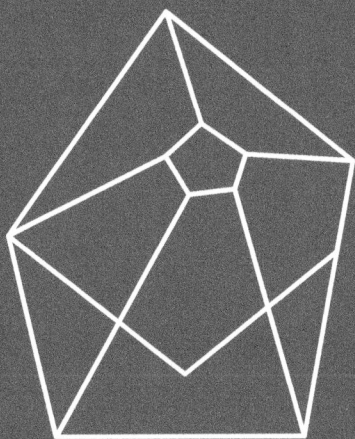

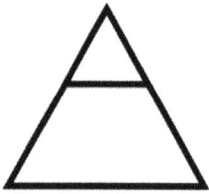

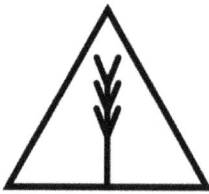

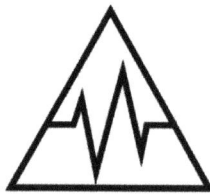

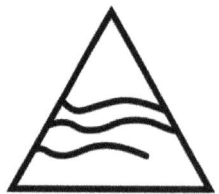

GCW PUBLISHING HOUSE

www.ingramcontent.com/pod-product-compliance
Lightning Source LLC
Chambersburg PA
CBHW041213030426
42336CB00023B/3330